The POTENT Male

Introduction by
William H. Masters, M.D.,
co-founder of the
Masters & Johnson
Institute

IRWIN GOLDSTEIN, M.D.
& LARRY ROTHSTEIN

Regenesis
Cycle
Publishing
Inc.

ISBN: 1-56852-063-8

Contents

———— ◆ ————

———— ◆ ————

———— ◆ ————

To Sue, the most special teacher, listener, friend and lover. And to Bryan, Lauren and Andrew, our beautiful, inspirational joy. I LOVE YOU ALL.

— Irwin

About the Authors

Irwin Goldstein, M.D.

Dr. Goldstein is a leading researcher and clinician in the field of impotence. He holds a bachelor's degree in engineering from Brown University with an honors thesis in biomedical engineering. In 1975, he graduated from McGill University Medical School, Montreal, Quebec, Canada, his hometown.

Dr. Goldstein is a Professor of Urology at Boston University School of Medicine. In 1988, he hosted and chaired the International Society of Impotence Research's biennial international meeting in Boston. In 1992 he was a member of the National Institutes of Health Impotence Consensus Development Panel and Conference in Bethesda, Maryland. In 1994 he participated in the largest epidemiologic study of impotence in the community since Kinsey, the Massachusetts Male Aging Study. Dr. Goldstein has been continuously funded for basic science impotence research at the National Institutes of Health since 1980. He has won numerous honors and awards for research in impotence including the Jack Lapides award and the American Urological Association Clinical Research Prize. Dr. Goldstein pioneered the "dynamic infusion cavernosometry and cavernosography" diagnostic technique to determine the exact nature of a man's erectile dysfunction, as well as several vascular reconstructive procedures, including penile revascularization, to restore natural potency in impotent patients.

He has published over 150 papers, chapters and reviews on the topic of impotence, including ones in the prestigious *New England Journal of Medicine, Journal of the American Medical Association, American Journal of Physiology* and *Journal of Urology.* He has also co-edited *Male Sexual Dysfunction* (Little, Brown, 1983) with R. J. Krane and M. B. Siroky. He has been featured in CBS's "The Body Human," ABC's "Good Morning America" and has appeared in several popular magazines and newspapers, including *Time, U.S. News and World Report* and the *Wall Street Journal.*

Dr. Goldstein now lives in Milton, Massachusetts with his wife, Sue, and their three children, Bryan, Lauren and Andrew.

Larry Rothstein

Larry Rothstein has a doctorate in education from Harvard University. He has previously co-authored *Minding the Body, Mending the Mind* (Addison-Wesley, 1988); *Dog Tales* (Warner, 1988); and *Conquering Shyness* (Putnam, 1989).

Contributors and Consultants

William H. Masters, M.D.

Co-chairman of the Board of the Masters & Johnson Institute, St. Louis, Missouri

Professor of Clinical Obstetrics and Gynecology, Washington University School of Medicine, St. Louis, Missouri

Lecturer in Human Sexuality in Psychiatry, Washington University School of Medicine, St. Louis, Missouri

Co-author with Virginia Johnson, D.Sc. (Hon.) of the landmark texts *Human Sexual Response* (Little, Brown, 1966) and *Human Sexual Inadequacy* (Little, Brown, 1970), and of many subsequent books. Their most recent book, with Robert Kolodny, is *Crisis: Heterosexual Behavior in the Age of AIDS* (Grove Press, 1988).

Alma Dell Smith, Ph.D.

Director of the Biobehavioral Treatment Center, Brookline, Massachusetts

Assistant Research Professor in Medicine (Psychology), Boston University School of Medicine, Boston

Director of Psychological Services, Woman's Health Group of Evans Medical Foundation, Boston University Medical Center

Mark L. Elliott, Ph.D.

Clinical Director, Masters & Johnson Institute, St. Louis, Missouri

Diplomate, American Board of Sexology

Robert J. Krane, M.D.

Professor and Chairman, Department of Urology, Boston University School of Medicine

Terry Payton, R.N., B.S.

Clinical Coordinator, Department of Urology, University Hospital, Boston

K. M. Rivard

Freelance writer

Illustrators

Lori Messenger

Biomedical Illustrator, Boston University School of Medicine

Scott Williams

Medical Illustrator, Boston University School of Medicine

Foreword

Over the last several years, the urological subspecialty of impotence has undergone enormous advancement. Progress has been especially striking in basic research on penile erections and in the diagnosis and treatment of erectile problems. *The Potent Male* offers the general reader a lucid explanation of these findings, both from the lab and the examining room.

In the laboratory, we have applied standard techniques of vascular experimentation to the study of potency. This has added greatly to our understanding of the basic nerve and blood-vessel physiology of the penile erection.

Chapters 1 and 2 of *The Potent Male* provide readers with an excellent introduction to impotence and male anatomy. The anatomy of the penis, and the neural, vascular, hormonal and psychological factors involved in an erection are treated in close detail with excellent illustrations.

Specifically, chapter 2 also identifies the three different aspects of the erection process —*initiating, filling* and *storing*— and how erectile problems may now be classified according to which of these mechanisms are compromised.

One indication of our new comprehension of the physiology of potency is our understanding of the connection between the state of the penis, in terms of its being erect or flaccid, and the "tone" (relaxed or contracted) of the smooth-muscle erection tissue of the penis. Under normal conditions this tone is controlled by a complex interaction of factors involving both nerves and blood vessels. Drugs have now been developed that relax the smooth-muscle tissue of the penis and initiate the development of an erection. Conversely, drugs that contract this tissue cause the penis to return to the nonerect state.

What does all of this mean for the impotent patient? For one thing, it signals our increased ability to distinguish erectile problems due to physical disease or injury from those with psychological origins. Furthermore, it means we are increasingly able to pinpoint which part of the erection process is affected.

In order to derive such specific knowledge of patients' problems, newer diagnostic techniques have been developed. These tests are performed on the penis in the erect state, an achievement that was neither routine nor predictable several years ago. In chapters 3 through 8, all of which present extensive patient stories, the gamut of diagnostic tests and treatments available today is discussed and reviewed. Chapter 9 looks forward to the future.

Marked progress has been made in the available therapies for the treatment of patients with erection problems. One of the most innovative medical treatments has been the self-injection of drugs into the erection chamber. These drugs relax the penile smooth-muscle tissue and induce erection. Chapter 6 tells the story of a couple who continue to deal successfully with the problem of impotence by utilizing injection therapy. Patients, as well as part-ners who may be interested in this treatment, will find a useful dis-cussion of the medical issues, as well as descriptions of the actual drugs and techniques used in this therapy.

Vascular reconstructive surgery for the impotent patient is one of the most innovative of the surgical treatments. Dr. Goldstein, a leader in the field of arterial reconstruction for impotence, has shown the ability to successfully restore erections in selected patients with impotence. Chapters 4 and 5 detail the case histories of two men who have undergone vascular reconstructive surgery in order to improve the quality of their erections. The chapters include explanations of the new surgical techniques and which patients are most likely to benefit from their use.

The availability of penile implants in the 1970s was probably the single most important event in the development of impotence treatment as a subspeciality of urology. Implants continue to undergo modification and design development, with several new hydraulic and nonhydraulic prostheses introduced in the last sev-eral years. Chapter 7 follows a couple whose lives were genuinely improved by the husband's penile implantation surgery. The chapter explores the features of different implants, how implant design has changed since the 1970s and the importance of tailor-ing patient expectations to the reality of implants.

As the title of chapter 1, *Impotence–the Last Taboo*, suggests, impo-tence treatment has too long been a forbidden topic. *The Potent Male* succeeds in providing explanation and insight into many of the newer developments in research, diagnosis and therapy for this problem. The presentation of this new information in such a readable and instructive format may provide invaluable assistance to the many individuals, couples and families who suffer, usually without such knowledge, from this common problem.

Robert J. Krane, M.D.
Professor and Chairman, Department of Urology
Boston University School of Medicine
University Hospital, Boston

Preface

The concept of a state-of-the-art medical book for the general reader on the topic of potency and impotence evolved after the publication of an interview I gave on the subject to a Boston newspaper.

I had no experience in writing for people outside the health-care field, but I knew that the patients I was seeing who had problems with their potency were often frustrated and embarrassed by their disorder. Moreover, many patients had misinformation about their condition. I realized that a book describing the mechanisms of erection and the advances in treating erection problems would be useful to the millions of men suffering from varying degrees of impotence.

The book I envisioned would enable the general reader to gain a realistic perspective on the latest information about impotence research and treatment.

And so *The Potent Male* was born and has reached all its expectations. This book encourages straight talk about the common and treatable problem of impotence. It teaches you the new scientific information on how the body produces an erection and how that process may be sabotaged by disease, injury, lifestyle and aging. The new methods of diagnosis of erection problems and the many new choices for treatment are fully discussed.

This book is not intended to substitute for the advice of a qualified urologist, but rather to lead you to one, armed with all the information you need to discuss your problem and make the best decision about whether to undergo treatment, and if so, what kind.

Irwin Goldstein, M.D.
Professor of Urology
Boston University School of Medicine

Acknowledgments

I would like to thank the many people who are responsible for molding this complex project into *The Potent Male*.

My patients are the ones who encouraged me, who provided the motivation, inspiration and insight to write this book. To my patients, especially those who gave of their time, effort and privacy to participate in this book, I thank you and pledge persistence in the research efforts of this troublesome, yet fascinating, medical problem.

I would like to thank all those individuals who have encouraged and supported my research work, initially in biomedical engineering at Brown University, and subsequently in medicine at McGill University. At Boston University School of Medicine, Carl A. Olsson, M.D., former Professor and Chairman of the Department of Urology, stimulated and encouraged me to perform urologic research during my residency training years. Robert J. Krane, M.D., Professor and present Chairman of the Department of Urology, has been my urologic mentor in impotence research. I am indebted to him for introducing me to the field and for continually supporting me in all aspects since.

Mike B. Siroky, M.D., Professor of Urology, both associate and advisor, provided invaluable assistance and direction during research training both in impotence and in neuro-urology. Herbert H. Wotiz, Ph.D., Professor of Biochemistry and Research Professor of Urology, and my father-in-law, has generously provided the combined gifts of basic science laboratory research experience and caring advice. Iñigo Saenz de Tejada, Associate Research Professor of Urology and previous director of the Urological Research Laboratory, began his involvement in impotence research in our laboratory as a medical student in 1982. His dedication, commitment and innovation in the basic science research of impotence is unparalleled and has already resulted in numerous outstanding discoveries and publications. He is fast becoming recognized as a leading researcher in impotence.

I would like to thank the members of the Urologic Research Laboratory at the Boston University School of Medicine for their outstanding work: Kazem Azadzoi, M.D., Abdul Traish, Ph.D., Richard Cohen, M.D., Robert Moreland, Ph.D., Sandeep Gupta, Ph.D., Jennifer Daley and Jeri McGrath-Cerqua. I would also like to recognize the support of Dean Aram Chobanian, M.D., for our research efforts within Boston University School of Medicine. I would like to thank Ronald Mortara, M.D., for teaching me microsurgical skills, Alan Greenfield, M.D., for his outstanding radiologic contributions in impotence, Gina DeGravio for her skill and enthusiasm in media relations, Edward Spatz, M.D., Chairman of the Department of Surgery, and Richard Egdahl, M.D., Director of the Boston University Medical Center, for their unyielding encouragement.

In addition, I wish to recognize the support and encouragement of our research work in impotence by the National Institute of Diabetes, Digestive Diseases and Kidney (NIDDK) of the National Institutes of Health (NIH). The initial Clinical Investigator Award in 1980 and the subsequent research grants in impotence have provided the long-term funding necessary to obtain the important health information on impotence. In particular, I wish to thank Charles H. Rodgers, M.D., previous Director of the Urology Program, Leroy M. Nyberg, Jr., M.D., present Director of the Urology Program, and Gary Striker, M.D., Director, Division of Kidney, Urological and Hematologic Diseases.

I would like to acknowledge the members of the New England Male Reproductive Center at the University Hospital for all their support in the clinical aspects of impotence: Richard K. Babayan, M.D., associate and ally from the residency training years to the associate professor years; Terry Payton, R.N., B.S., nurse clinician, specialist in impotence, colleague and co-worker in the field with whom numerous of the clinical achievements have been developed; Laurie McCann, who has helped maintain organization in my life; and Karen Cooper, who initially coordinated the clinic and, as administrative assistant, has managed to maintain the department as a cohesive unit.

I am truly grateful to the urologists who have trained with me — Harin Padma-Nathan, M.D., Tim Roddy, M.D., Jocelyne Tessier, M.D., Fred Levine, M.D., Barbara Gasior, M.D., Alan D. Seftel, M.D., Dimitrios G. Hatzichristou, M.D., Eduardo Bertero, M.D., Edoardo S. Pescatori, M.D., Guido Basile, M.D., Ajay Nehra, M.D., Martin Bastuba, M.D., and Larry Hakim, M.D. I am indebted to many friends and colleagues who perform research and contribute to the field. There is not enough space to mention all their names, but the organizations and societies to which they belong include the American Urological Association, the American Foundation for Urologic Diseases, the Society for the Study of Impotence, the International Society for Impotence Research, the National Kidney Foundation, the Urologic and Reproductive Biology Forums at the American College of Surgery and the Humana Impotence Research Study Group. Their outstanding contributions are listed in the extensive bibliography at the end of this book.

Although the idea for the book was sound, the writing could not have taken place without the expertise of many individuals.

I thank Ken Rivard, a gifted creative writer who worked with Larry and me, and with whom it was a genuine pleasure to exchange ideas. I appreciate the effort by Alma Dell Smith, Ph.D., a colleague in the field since the early 1980s, for taking the time from her busy work schedule to act as psychological consultant for the book. I am honored to have had the participation of both William H. Masters, M.D. and Robert J. Krane, M.D., who wrote the introduction and foreword, respectively. Both individuals have also contributed immensely to the field of impotence and sexual dysfunction.

I thank Lori Messenger and Scott Williams for their talent in producing remarkably effective and understandable illustrations for the text.

I would like to acknowledge my parents, brother and sister. My mother, Anne, taught me lessons in humor, sensitivity and caring. My father, Sol, taught me lessons in perseverance, pride and family. Their ethics — family first, work hard and play hard — remain vital sustaining forces in my life. My brother Myron is a classic big brother, always there when I need advice and support. My sister Betty is an invaluable source of needed caring and love.

Finally, I would like to give special appreciation to my own family. I would like to thank my children Bryan, Lauren and Andrew. Their constant thirst for knowledge and vitality for life continuously inspire me. My wife Sue and I, from our college days to the present, have taken on numerous challenges together. Writing this book was no different. Her unsung involvement extended from confidante to editor and everything in between. Clearly this book could not have been created without her, and for that I can only say I love her more.

— *Irwin Goldstein*

Introduction

In the last forty years, the burgeoning demand for adequate treatment of the many-faceted problems of human sexual dysfunction has stimulated the growth of a new, loosely structured specialty in the health-care field.

Unfortunately, academic education in the biological and behavioral sciences does not provide the training necessary for the professional who desires to treat human sexual inadequacy. Today's medical schools do not give students sufficient exposure to the basic sciences of psychology or sociology. By the same token, doctoral training in the behavioral sciences rarely includes in-depth education in the biological sciences, such as anatomy or physiology, or even a superficial exposure to such clinical areas as endocrinology, pharmacology, urology or gynecology.

Certainly, it is true that sexual dysfunction can be primarily caused by either psychological or biological factors. But it is also true that in many instances the therapist encounters a combination of both psychological and biological problems when evaluating and treating male or female sexual inadequacy. This is particularly true when the therapist has to deal with the complex problems of the sexually impotent man.

When a new health-care discipline emerges, most professionals in the field have to gain expertise through on-the-job training. Inevitably, many "therapeutic loopholes" are created by this type of training. There are many therapists now treating psychological problems of the impotent male who have not become adequately oriented to the specific details of penile anatomy, or even more important, to the physiology of penile erection. Also, many penile implants are inserted either because of inadequate psychosexual evaluation or because surgical skills are not adequate to reverse the vascular problem that has created the man's impotence. One would hope that in the remaining decade of this century, these professional inadequacies would not only be identified, but to a large extent, resolved.

The other area in which progress must be made is in the keeping of adequate follow-up statistics for different methods used in treating impotence. Certainly, the major treatment centers in this country have this inherent responsibility, yet few have responded to such an important educational opportunity. Only one center has maintained and made available five-year follow-up statistics for the treatment of psychologically caused impotence, and follow-up information regarding penile implant surgery has not been made routinely available five to ten years after the surgical procedure was performed.

The incidences of equipment failure, of the need for repeat surgery and of rejection by female partners must be thoroughly analyzed.

Furthermore, we must determine whether there are long-term negative consequences of frequent penile injections of papaverine and phentolamine. Maintaining and publishing detailed follow-up statistics encourages self-criticism by doctors and other therapists, without which "professional maturity of the field" is delayed or perhaps never attained.

In short, during the last forty years, therapy for human sexual dysfunction — with its psychological, medical and surgical branches — has grown "like Topsy." During the next decade, these healthcare specialties must come of age. *The Potent Male* may provide the impetus and chart a pathway for the different professionals involved in such therapy to move together into the twenty-first century. In this book, the causes of male impotence are given detailed consideration from both biological and psychological viewpoints. Currently accepted therapeutic techniques are presented in detail. Most important, the frequently expressed underlying theme of the book is that adequate diagnosis and treatment of the impotent male usually requires the services of professionals from more than one discipline, who can provide treatment from more than one perspective.

William H. Masters, M.D.
Masters & Johnson Institute
St. Louis, Missouri

CHAPTER 1

Impotence – The Last Taboo

"He was sexually inadequate ... a scared man, a weak man, timid, afraid–*Impotent! Impotent! Impotent!*" screams the defense lawyer in the 1987 movie *From the Hip*. The lawyer is hoping to associate impotence with inadequacy and thereby prove his client is innocent of a brutal murder. The strategy backfires; the defendant is so enraged by his lawyer's statements that he leaps from his chair, brandishing the murder weapon. No one gets away with calling him impotent–not his lawyer, and certainly not the woman he murdered! In this movie, a pedantic, ineffectual college professor bludgeons to death a prostitute who threatens to reveal his secret–his impotence. The suggestion is that he chose to commit murder rather than allow anyone, including himself, to face this truth. *From the Hip* exemplifies all the old falsehoods about sexual impotence–that it is associated with general inadequacy, neurosis, character flaws, even outright insanity. Is it any wonder so many impotent men have kept silent about this problem?

The latest estimates are that 20–30 million American men are impotent–most of them for basic physical reasons related to vascular disease, injuries or aging. But, for most of them, impotence is still a source of shame and humiliation. It's been called "the last taboo." Fear and ignorance attend its discussion–when it gets discussed at all.

Many of the men I've treated over the last fifteen years have told me that they couldn't tell anyone about the problems they were having with their lack of potency. They were ashamed. They were afraid their manhood would be called into question if they confessed they couldn't perform in the bedroom.

When we fear something, we tend to keep silent about it, or we cover up our fear with a mask of disdain or contempt. Movies, jokes and popular culture reinforce such negative attitudes. It isn't surprising that few men have sought treatment for their impotence. Not that treatment, until recently, has been all that great.

"WITCHCRAFT"

References to impotence have appeared in literature and medical writings since the beginning of recorded history, with various theories concerning its origin.

The ancient Greek physician Hippocrates, often described as the "Father of Medicine," knew of the problem and attributed it to preoccupation with business or to an unattractive wife. Lacking our present knowledge of erectile physiology, he didn't have the whole picture.

Throughout history, treatment of impotence has rarely risen above the level of witchcraft. In the nineteenth century, it was found that castrated roosters no longer achieved erections, but that after their testicles were surgically restored, the erections returned. This discovery inaugurated decades of glandular extracts and fake testicular potions guaranteed to rejuvenate "lost manhood."

Surgical solutions to improve hormonal balance were equally ineffective. In 1918, it was reported that "youth could be renewed" by grafting the cells of monkey testicles into men. In the 1920s, some urologists were advocating surgery that interrupts the movement of sperm away from the testicle as a cure for impotence. (Such surgery, called a *vasectomy*, is now performed as a method of permanent contraception.) Even transplantation of human testicles enjoyed a certain vogue for a time as a treatment for impotence.

The grain of truth at the heart of some of these treatments is that hormones produced in the testicles *do* have an effect on erections. But that effect is far from completely understood (see *Low Testosterone and Other Hormonal Disorders*, page 157). In any case, modern research has shown that most impotence is apparently *not* related to hormone deficiencies. Hormone-based treatments should be used only by those impotent patients who have a documented hormonal abnormality.

Since the 1930s, surgeons have been experimenting with various kinds of devices that artificially stiffen the penis and enable the patient to have intercourse. Since the 1970s, these devices have become very reliable and effective, as you'll see in chapter 7. But, the drawback in this kind of surgery is that it forever closes the door on any chance of restoring a man's own erectile physiology.

Even today, knowledge of the dramatic advances in impotence research, diagnosis and treatment have yet to be widely disseminated.

Some doctors still place a misguided faith in hormone supplements and use them for most patients with impotence. And, as recently as ten years ago, many reputable medical authorities still believed that only 10 percent of impotence had a physical cause. The remaining 90 percent of patients were thought to have psychological problems that caused their difficulties—and they often underwent years of psychotherapy to no avail.

We now suspect that as much as 80 to 90 percent of impotence may be associated with underlying *physical* abnormalities related to "vascular risk factors" (such as smoking and too much fat and cholesterol in the diet), injuries (automobile accidents, sports-related injuries, childhood accidents and so on), disease (particularly diabetes and multiple sclerosis) and the changes in tissue associated with aging. Perhaps 10 to 20 percent of impotent men are impotent for *solely* psychological reasons and have no physical abnormalities in their erectile mechanisms.

That is not to say that psychological factors are unimportant. The majority of impotent men with physical abnormalities interfering with function to a varying extent experience some degree of humiliation, frustration, anger, fear, guilt or depression, all of which contribute to a worsening of the problem. My point, which I hope this book demonstrates, is that *physical factors resulting in changes in the erectile mechanism—that is, changes in hardness of the erection and sustaining ability of the erection—are much more common than previously believed.* More often than not, it is a physical problem that is the primary cause of erection difficulties. Psychological factors usually occur as a secondary response to the underlying primary physical problem. Longstanding impotence is rarely "all in the head."

NEW ANSWERS

Impotence is just now becoming a "hot" topic. In the past, with so few men willing to admit to the problem, there was little public pressure for treatment. Since then, especially in the last ten years, we have made significant headway toward understanding the causes of impotence, how to diagnose the exact problem and, finally, how to treat it.

After I completed urology residency training, I was fortunate to receive a National Institutes of Health research grant. This particular clinical investigator award was designed to allow me to study energy losses in the urinary stream. Our research didn't lead directly to any breakthroughs concerning energy losses, but we did notice that every time we stimulated the nerves of an animal's bladder, he got an erection. After we completed the urinary research, we decided to develop the animal model further in order to study the basic physiology of erections. My subsequent medical research has been exclusively in the field of impotence. This is, in part, an outgrowth of my earlier training in biomedical engineering and later years as a physician and medical researcher.

Technical advances have happened quickly. Just a few years ago, for example, when I wanted to measure the blood pressure in a patient's penile arteries, I had to rely on a blood-pressure cuff that was actually designed for children's arms—not adult penises. We were also forced to rely on measurements of blood pressures in a nonerect penis instead of measuring blood pressure when it really counts—during the process of erection.

Once we improved our equipment and our testing, we began to answer our questions about circulation in the penis and to suspect that blocked arteries affected potency. It was only natural that the next step would be the development of surgical procedures to improve blood flow to the penis.

In our own institution, Boston University Medical Center, the first ten cases of "bypass surgery" for blocked penile arteries were failures—nobody's erection capacity improved. All the men in this first group of patients were between fifty and sixty years old, and all had significant problems with their blood vessels from years of smoking, high cholesterol and hypertension.

Then, a twenty-year-old patient with impotence was referred to the clinic. He was found to have a very low blood pressure in the main artery of his penis, and we suspected he had an arterial blockage. We sent him to the radiology department for X rays using dye. The radiologists initially declined to do the X rays—they said twenty-year-olds shouldn't have arterial blockages! They didn't want to expose him to the radiation necessary to do the test. Eventually, though, they did agree to perform the X-ray study, and there it was—significant blockage in this young man's penile arteries, the result of a previously fractured pelvis from an auto accident. We operated on him, bypassing the blockages, and his potency was restored.

The success of that operation taught us to distinguish between blockages that are localized in a few areas and blockages that are widely scattered through the whole arterial network. As you might suspect, localized blockages are often the result of accidental injury to the pelvic area; diffuse blockages are associated with smoking, a diet excessively rich in fat and cholesterol, or aging. We can now do bypass surgery for the localized blockages, but other kinds of treatments seem to be better for the more diffuse kind.

We can't yet restore the natural erectile physiology of all impotent men, but we can restore their potency in virtually all cases. Later in this book, I'll describe in detail the new therapies we use to accomplish this goal.

Since most people haven't the vaguest idea of how the body produces an erection, much of the information in this book will be new, and at first you may find it strange and unfamiliar. Please be patient. I'm trying to map out a territory previously unknown to many of you, and many of the place names will be unfamiliar. Chapter 2 explains in detail how erections work. You will read how the body's muscle tissue, nerves and blood vessels cooperate to produce an erection. You will also learn how disease, injury, lifestyle and aging may sabotage this process and how these problems can be treated and even sometimes prevented. Later chapters examine the role of sex therapy, different kinds of surgeries and other treatments for impotence. Chapter 8 addresses the special concerns of men with diabetes, spinal-cord injuries, cancer and other conditions that can affect potency.

HOW TO GET
THE BEST POSSIBLE TREATMENT

My hope is that, having once examined the "map" that is drawn in this book, you will then seek out a guide–a urologist who specializes in impotence treatment. Even if you think that your problem is "all in your head," it is important that you eliminate the possibility of any physical causes for your impotence. Once that concern is gone, a sex therapist or other counselor can help you explore the emotional issues that interfere with a healthy sex life.

———— ◆ ————

There are many ways to find a urologist. Your family doctor is the first person to ask for a referral. Specify that you want a urologist who specializes in the treatment of impotence. The white pages listings of local university medical schools are another good resource. Call their urology departments, outline your case and ask for referrals. Most states also have medical societies for each specialty. The society should have a list of urologists who treat impotence.

If you aren't comfortable with any of the above suggestions, there's another alternative. Support groups such as Impotence Anonymous usually have the names of the best doctors in the area for dealing with impotence. Their encouragement and support also help many men overcome their resistance to talking about what they feel is a humiliating problem. Once you get the name of a doctor, don't hesitate to call and ask a few preliminary questions over the phone. After all, you're entrusting the most intimate part of your life to his or her care.

In many cases, the urologist will be at the head of a team of specialists that you will encounter during diagnosis and treatment of your problem. It is important that you find a urologist who is caring, well informed and knowledgeable about impotence and the broader issues of human sexuality. He or she should be certified by the American Board of Urology and should keep abreast of the latest developments in the field through continuing medical education. (For a guide to the steps a urologist should follow in doing an evaluation for impotence, see *What Happens at the Urologist's Office* below). He or she should be willing to refer you to other specialists if initial testing uncovers problems that fall outside of the urologist's expertise. The other members of the team might include the following specialists.

An edocrinologist specializes in the diagnosis of hormonal problems. The male hormone *testosterone* (see *The Testicles*, page 14 and *Low Testosterone and Other Hormonal Disorders*, page 157) is sometimes involved in the diagnosis and treatment of impotence. Occasionally, other hormones are used in the treatment of impotence.

A neurologist specializes in treating disorders of the nervous system, an important consideration for men with a history of spinalcord or other nerve injury or disease, alcoholism or diabetes (see chapter 8). Neurologists can conduct tests that tell whether the nerves to and from the penis are communicating with the spinal cord and brain.

A psychiatrist or psychologist specializes in the emotional and mental aspects of impotence diagnosis and treatment. Almost all impotence, regardless of its source, has psychological effects. A therapist can help a couple clarify their thinking when deciding among various treatment options. After treatment, he or she can also help a couple make a smooth adjustment to a restored love life (see chapter 3 for a further explanation of the role of sex therapy and counseling.)

An internist or family physician addresses the broader medical issues that affect a man's health, including his potency. He or she addresses the patient's smoking, high blood pressure, high cholesterol, diabetes or heart disease. Reducing these factors, through medication or changes in lifestyle, may stop the progress of an erection problem.

WHAT HAPPENS AT THE UROLOGIST'S OFFICE

There are at the present time no certifying examinations for urologists in impotence diagnosis and management, no board to certify impotence specialists and no objective means of identifying impotence experts among urologists. Reading this book should help you evaluate whether or not your urologist has a thorough grounding in impotence treatment, as should your experience in his or her office. Though no two doctors will conduct a history and physical exam in exactly the same way, the following steps should be covered in a urologist's evaluation for impotence:

1. A urologist will begin with your medical history. You should tell him or her about any serious illness, past or present, even if it's not bothering you right now and there seem to be no lasting effects. You should also be sure to mention any surgery or injuries you've suffered, especially to the back, pelvic or perineal (crotch) area. You should also talk about any medications you are taking and about your use of alcohol, tobacco and other drugs.

2. Your sexual history comes next. Although these questions are intensely personal, your answers provide the urologist with information critical to making an accurate diagnosis. He or she will probably ask you about the rigidity and sustaining capability of your erections during intercourse, during masturbation and upon awakening in the morning. He or she will want to know how your erections differ from those you've had in the past, including when and under what circumstances you first noticed any changes. You may be asked to describe your sexual activity, especially your present and past frequency of intercourse. Do you have orgasms, and can you ejaculate? If you have difficulty in either area, it's important to describe how often the problem occurs and under exactly what circumstances.

3. A physical exam will follow the discussion of your sexual history. The exam will focus special attention on the reflexes, sensations and pulses in your legs and pelvic area and take a complete look at your penis and testicles to check for any abnormalities. The complete workup for impotence may also include blood tests to determine hormone levels.

4. Your medical and sexual histories and your physical exam and lab results will help the urologist determine which, if any, underlying medical conditions may be causing your problem. Depending on these results, the urologist may require further testing. He or she may want to study the pattern of your sleep erections and may ask you to undergo more sophisticated tests. Some tests help determine the location of arterial blockages, while others measure whether excessive amounts of blood are flowing away from the penis during the erection process. All of these tests are explained in subsequent chapters, but you are entitled to an explanation from your urologist during your office visit.

5. It may take several visits, and even a consultation or two with another specialist, but the urologist should eventually give you a diagnosis. He or she may provide you with additional written or visual material in order to make sure that you understand your condition. He or she should then explain the various treatment options, including what will happen if the first course of action doesn't work out.

6. He or she should ask you to return for a follow-up examination to see how you are doing.

STRAIGHT TALK

In the following pages, you will encounter several histories of men of different backgrounds and ages that I have diagnosed and treated since 1980. I've encouraged them to discuss their sexual histories and experiences at length. Names and significant details like occupations and hometowns have been changed to protect the identity of each man. Each of their stories is followed by a commentary explaining how I came to my diagnosis, how the man was treated, how he's doing today and how the field has evolved since his treatment. Many of the chapters also feature an analysis of the psychological dimension of the patient's impotence by Dr. Alma Dell Smith, an experienced psychologist and sex therapist to whom I refer many of my patients.

It is my hope that this book will encourage some straight talk about impotence. I want you to see impotence for what it is—a treatable condition, like heart disease or a broken leg. Few problems are so amenable to treatment, yet are so frequently untreated, because of shame, guilt, fear—or the simple lack of understanding. If I've managed to lift the veil that still covers the discussion and treatment of impotence for many people, I've done my job.

CHAPTER 2

Erections

- **How They Work**
- **How They Sometimes Don't Work**
- **What Can Be Done About Them**

On the corner of my desk, within easy reach of a visitor's chair, sits a well-thumbed volume on pelvic anatomy. With its graphic multi-color illustrations and jawbreaker terminology, the book is quite plainly written for surgeons, yet I refer my patients to it often. I want them to understand exactly what we're talking about. If I diagnose an abnormality with blood storing, or blocked arteries, I want them to know where to find the anatomical problem.

In my experience, most men know more about the workings of the combustion engine than about the dynamics of their own sex life. Women tend to be considerably better informed about themselves—and they share information. Even modest bookstores have at least one shelf devoted to gynecological information, and large bookstores often have three or four times that number. Accessible answers to questions about their sexuality have become tantamount to a political right for women. I don't think an equivalent right—or shelf of books—exists for men.

One of my patients, in his mid-thirties, remarked that for years he'd suspected something was wrong with his erections. Suspected, but wasn't sure. Sometimes he would get an erection that would allow him and his wife to begin intercourse, but after a few minutes of thrusting, he would begin to lose hardness in his penis, and then his erection would just melt away. Almost fifteen years elapsed before he found help.

Looking back, the patient recalled the advice of his family doctor: "My doctor told me that he had the same 'problem,' but that it was perfectly normal—which it wasn't. What could I, as a patient, do? You don't talk to your friends about how their penises behave. How are you supposed to know if your erection is normal? It's such a forbidden topic. I would have felt a lot better—at least I'd have known something was wrong—if I'd had the chance to read about what a normal erection is like."

———— ◆ ————

This chapter is a short course in the anatomy and physiology of an erection, an effort to provide the information my patient so sorely missed. Here's what I cover:

- the male reproductive system, with a close look at the penis and testicles
- the role of the autonomic nervous system
- the biomechanics of an erection
- the potency spectrum
- *initiating, filling* and *storing*—the erection problem areas, with some of their causes
- the different options for treatment
- a word about prevention of impotence.

If you're a man who thinks he might have a problem with impotence—or a woman who suspects her husband or lover might have one—you should take some time to inform yourself about how erections work, how they sometimes don't work and how they can be treated today.

Anatomy

The following anatomical discussion may seem overly detailed, but it will help you understand how and why the different components of your system work together—or fail to work. As you read, it will help you to refer to the illustrations on pages 11, 12 and 13.

THE PENIS

Penis shapes and sizes vary widely among animals, reflecting some of the wilder adaptive techniques seen in nature. Penises are corkscrew-shaped in pigs; in kangaroos they have double heads (which makes an ideal match for female kangaroos, since they have double vaginas). The shaft of the penis in most mammals contains a slender bone, which keeps the penis in a constant state of semierection. Man,

Anatomy of Penis and Surrounding Organs

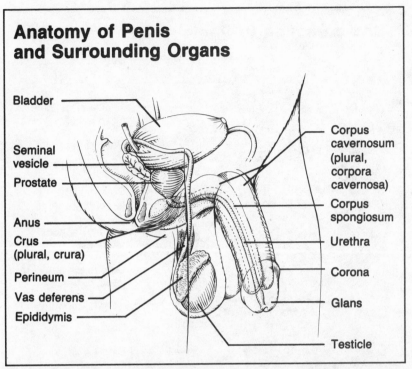

Bladder

Seminal vesicle

Prostate

Anus

Crus (plural, crura)

Perineum

Vas deferens

Epididymis

Corpus cavernosum (plural, corpora cavernosa)

Corpus spongiosum

Urethra

Corona

Glans

Testicle

The penis consists of two balloon-like cylinders, each one called a corpus caver-nosum or erection chamber, and a third cylinder that surrounds the urethra, called the corpus spongiosum (area inside dotted line). One half of the penis is hidden; it extends almost all the way to the anus, and attaches to the pelvis. The portion of the penis that attaches to the pelvis is called the crus (plural, crura), and there is one on each side of the penis.

however, has no such bone. His erections are achieved by vascular mechanics—i.e., by the penis filling with and storing blood—and are thus temporary occurrences.

In its flaccid state, the human penis is more or less round, a soft cylinder of spongy tissue. One half of the human penis is actually hidden; it extends inside the body almost all the way to the anus, where it attaches to the undersurface of the pelvis (see illustration above). The concealed part of the penis is called the *crus* (plural, *crura*). Despite its placement inside the body, it is extremely vulnerable to injury. In later chapters we'll see how specific pelvic injuries can damage this area, sometimes resulting in impotence.

Anatomically, the penis is a "balloon," or rather two long balloons lying next to each other: two *corpora cavernosa* (Latin plural for "hollow bodies"), which are also called *erection chambers*. There is another, smaller chamber, the *corpus spongiosum* ("spongy body"), which sur-rounds the urinary passageway.

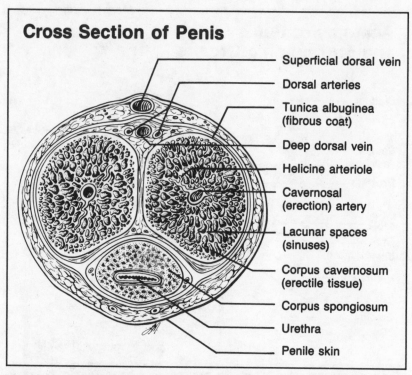

Cross Section of Penis

- Superficial dorsal vein
- Dorsal arteries
- Tunica albuginea (fibrous coat)
- Deep dorsal vein
- Helicine arteriole
- Cavernosal (erection) artery
- Lacunar spaces (sinuses)
- Corpus cavernosum (erectile tissue)
- Corpus spongiosum
- Urethra
- Penile skin

This view shows the corpora cavernosa, each surrounded by a tough, fibrous coat, the tunica albuginea. The cavernosa are filled with microscopic spaces called lacunar spaces or sinuses (shown by the white areas in the corpora cavernosa). The cavernosal, or erection artery, sends arterial blood to the lacunar spaces via smaller branches called the helicine arterioles.

The *tunica albuginea* (literally, the "white coat"), is a tough, fibrous tissue that surrounds both of the corpora cavernosa and provides a casing for the erectile tissue inside. The corpora cavernosa, or erectile chambers, are filled with erectile tissue that consists of microscopic chambers known as *lacunar spaces* or *sinuses*. When the penis is soft, the lacunar spaces are flattened, much like empty balloons, but during arousal, they swell with blood, stiffening, lengthening and expanding the separate corpora cavernosa until the penis becomes firm and erect.

The *corpus spongiosum,* on the underside of the penis, contains the *urethra.* The urethra has a dual function: It provides an outlet for urine from the bladder and a channel for semen during ejaculation. In a healthy man, urine and semen never enter the urethra at the same time.

The external end of the corpus spongiosum expands to form the acorn-shaped head of the penis, known as the *glans* (Latin for "acorn").

Cross Section of Penis with Expanded View of Smooth Muscle Surrounding a Lacunar Space (Sinus)

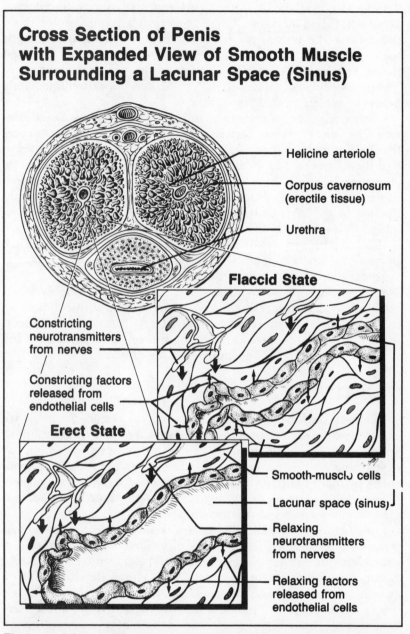

Helicine arteriole

Corpus cavernosum (erectile tissue)

Urethra

Flaccid State

Constricting neurotransmitters from nerves

Constricting factors released from endothelial cells

Erect State

Smooth-muscle cells

Lacunar space (sinus)

Relaxing neurotransmitters from nerves

Relaxing factors released from endothelial cells

The tone of the smooth muscle surrounding the lacunar spaces determines the amount of blood in the lacunar space and therefore is critical in the erection process. Nerves to the smooth muscle and factors from the endothelial cells that line the lacunar spaces control the tone of the smooth muscle—i.e., whether it is constricted or relaxed. In the flaccid state, the smooth-muscle tissue is constricted. In the erect state, it is relaxed.

A ridge around the base of the glans, especially prominent during arousal, is called the *corona* (Greek for "crown"). Immediately behind the corona, the skin of the penis extends outward and then folds back in on itself, completely covering the glans on uncircumcised males. This hood, or *foreskin,* can be rolled back to expose the glans. The glans, especially the corona and the band of skin immediately below it, is rich in sensory nerves.

Edgar Gregersen, in his wonderfully informative book, *Sexual Practices: The Story of Human Sexuality* (Franklin Watts, 1983), estimates that half of the world's males have been *circumcised*—that is, they've had their foreskins surgically removed. As a religious rite, circumcision can be traced back at least as far as the Egyptians, with some speculation that it was practiced even in the Stone Age. Until recently, doctors in the West routinely removed the foreskins of newborn males. This was prompted by a misguided belief that uncircumcised males ran a higher risk of cancer of the penis, a supposition since proven false, and a concern about cleanliness and protection against venereal disease and other infections.

As long as care is taken to clean the glans thoroughly when washing, men with foreskins run no higher risk of infection than those without. The presence or absence of a foreskin has no bearing on the ability to have an erection, nor on the sensitivity of the penis or the ability to become physically aroused.

THE TESTICLES

The most obvious of the male sexual organs besides the penis are the *testicles,* the storehouses for new sperm. The testicles both make sperm and supply 95 percent of the hormones responsible for developing and maintaining masculine characteristics. *Testosterone* is the primary male hormone, or *androgen*—literally, "man maker." (A very small amount of androgens are also produced by the adrenal glands, located right above the kidneys.)

Long before anyone knew about testosterone, people observed that if boys were castrated before puberty, they failed to develop masculine characteristics. During the seventeenth and eighteenth centuries, the European public's fascination with boys' choirs developed into a cultish adoration of *castrati,* deliberately castrated singers whose voices never deepened into the normal register of an adult man. But, an exquisitely high voice came at the cost of a masculine appearance, and commonly, but not always, of sexual desire.

We know that testosterone spurs sexual desire and influences the ability to have an erection. But, young boys, even male babies in the uterus, achieve erections in the virtual absence of testosterone (there is very little testosterone secreted by boys before puberty). And, some men who lose both their testicles through an accident or cancer, continue to have normal erections. The loss of a single testicle usually won't affect erections or desire.

So, it is unclear just how testosterone influences the process of erection. The relationship between testicle injury, testosterone levels and impotence is not nearly so straightforward as once thought.

If, after repeated testing, I find a patient has a consistently low level of testosterone, I refer him to our endocrinologist, who may then prescribe supplemental testosterone. In my own practice, however, I've found that the cause of the erection problem is rarely related to low hormone levels.

All the testosterone in the world won't cause an erection in a man who has a blocked artery or an abnormality in his blood-storage mechanism (discussed later in this chapter), which are the more common physical causes of erection problems.

A thin sack of skin and involuntary muscle, the *scrotum*, encloses the testicles in individual compartments. A second muscle, the *cremasteric muscle*, wraps around the connection of each testicle to the body. Both of these muscles draw the testicles close to the body.

As any man who has ever strolled from a warm beach into a freezing ocean will attest, the skin of the scrotum contracts into thick folds when exposed to a sudden drop in temperature; this helps insulate the testicles. For less well-understood reasons, the testicles also rise during states of fear or anger, and during arousal.

If you examine your testicles (see box below) you should feel a soft, raised ridge running alongside each testicle. This ridge is the *epididymis* (Greek for "at or near the testicle"), a place where new sperm

---

Examining Your Testicles

I encourage you to examine your testicles each time you shower or bathe. Roll each testicle between your fingers. It should feel soft and egg-shaped, and both testicles should be approximately the same size. Excessive manipulation should cause discomfort, leading to pain. Early warning signs of a tumor are lumpiness, hard nodules or the absence of pain when the testicle is pressed firmly. The presence of any of these symptoms should prompt an immediate examination by a urologist, who can perform further tests to check for a tumor. I emphasize such frequent self-exams because cancer of the testicle has a cure rate of virtually 100 percent when detected in its early stages.

mature. Each epididymis is a series of tiny, winding passages that provides an avenue out of the testicles for sperm.

The epididymis is a good example of the body's skill at miniaturization—uncoiled, each epididymis would stretch to be almost twenty feet long.

A narrow tube, the *vas deferens* ("vessel that carries away"), conveys sperm from each epididymis up through the pelvis into a widening of the vas called the *ampulla* ("little jar"), where sperm is stored.

THE SEMINAL VESICLES, PROSTATE AND COWPER'S GLANDS

Most of semen's bulk is a protective medium that enables sperm to survive their journey down the urethra and out through the penis. Sperm makes up only a minute fraction of semen's content. The far greater part is *seminal fluid*, from the *seminal vesicles*, and *prostatic fluid*, from the *prostate*. Men who undergo a *vasectomy* (sterilization surgery that prevents sperm from passing through the vas deferens) notice little or no change in the physical appearance of their semen, despite the fact that it no longer contains sperm, because it still contains seminal and prostatic fluids.

Underneath the prostate are a pair of glands shaped like thick dragonfly wings, the *seminal vesicles*, which produce the seminal fluid that mixes with the sperm to form semen. The seminal vesicles depend on hormones from the testicles for their activation; in a castrated man, the seminal vesicles wither away, and his semen, lacking seminal fluid, looks appreciably different.

A walnut-sized gland, the *prostate*, provides semen's third important ingredient, *prostatic fluid*. Unfortunately, as a man passes into his fifties, his prostate gland becomes increasingly vulnerable to infection, swelling and tumors. I recommend that after the age of forty-five, a man undergo a yearly prostatic examination.

Prostatic surgery, especially for cancer, long held a certain risk of impotence because an important nerve leading to the penis passes very close to the prostate. But recent surgical innovations have reduced the risk, and many younger men with confined tumors can now undergo a surgical removal of the entire prostate without a loss in their ability to achieve and sustain an erection.

During arousal you may have noticed a clear liquid oozing from the tip of your penis. A pair of glands on either side of the urethra, just forward of the prostate, sits on either side of the urethra. They're known as *Cowper's glands* and are about the size and shape of peas. It is believed they help lubricate the urethra during foreplay for the passage of semen during ejaculation.

Men sense the coming together of sperm and fluids from the seminal vesicles and prostate as a feeling that they're about to *ejaculate* (reach orgasm). Several distinct muscle groups in the pelvis and around the urethra cooperate to produce the powerful contractions that expel the semen out through the prostate and urethra. You may have noticed that muscles around the anus contract at the same time. This is because the same nerve feeds all three sets of muscles.

NERVES

A full discussion of the role of the nervous system in the functioning of male sexuality lies beyond the scope of this book. However, it's important to explain how different components of the nervous system affect your ability to become erect and have an orgasm.

Anatomists divide the body's neural network into the *central nervous system,* composed of the brain and spinal cord, and the *peripheral nervous system,* the complex bundles of fibers and receptors that transmit information and commands between the central nervous system and distant parts of the body.

If you imagine a large office building, with a central computer coordinating all of the building's various systems — electricity, heating, air conditioning, etc. — each of which is directly connected by wiring to the central computer, you have a good idea of the relationship between the brain and spinal cord and the peripheral nervous system. The central computer is analogous to the central nervous system (the brain and spinal cord); the connecting wires are analogous to the peripheral nervous system (the nerves that run between the brain and spinal cord and the rest of the body).

One part of the peripheral nervous system, the *autonomic nervous system,* deals with "involuntary" or "automatic" functions of the body. Breathing, heartbeat and digestion are examples of autonomic functions. So is your ability to have an erection and to have an orgasm.

Within the autonomic system itself (I promise, this is the final division) the nerves split again into the *sympathetic* and the *parasympathetic* system. Your emotional state determines which set of nerves operates at any given time.

During highly charged situations, the sympathetic system runs the show; the so-called "fight-or-flight" mechanism, when an animal has to decide whether to stand and fight an enemy or to flee, is under the sympathetic system's control. But during periods of relative calm, the parasympathetic system takes charge.

Generally speaking, the systems oppose each other. Imagine two groups of office workers, both of which are necessary to run a business. One group performs best if allowed to play rock 'n' roll in the background, but other workers prefer "easy listening," or no music at all. The rock 'n' rollers are analogous to the sympathetic system; the easy listeners to the parasympathetic. Each takes turns, or anarchy results.

In terms of function, the parasympathetic system is involved with the ability to get an erection, whereas the sympathetic system is involved with *detumescence* (getting soft) and maintaining you in the soft state.

The central nervous system also reflects the fact that erection and ejaculation are under separate controls. Since the nerves for ejaculation and erection are located in different parts of the spine, some men with impotence caused by nerve damage may have an ejaculation without an erection.

Biomechanics of an Erection

An erection works in a fashion remarkably similar to a *pneumatic device* such as a tire or balloon or a *hydraulic* device such as a waterbed; that is, a medium enters a previously low-pressure system and pressurizes and expands the space while being stored within the device.

An erection is a *hydraulic* system in which a liquid medium — blood — pressurizes and expands a previously low-pressure system.

When air is forced into a scuba tank, the air pressure inside the tank increases. When water is introduced into a waterbed, the water-bed expands and gets more firm. When blood flows into the penis, the penile blood pressure increases and the penis gets more firm.

The mechanics of an erection are deceptively simple — blood flows into the penis, is stored, and the penis expands until it becomes firm. Yet only within the last ten years have we begun to piece together the biochemical and physiological steps in this process. Even today, some of those steps have yet to be fully understood.

The important thing to realize is that the more we learn about each step, the greater will be our insight into the origin of each man's particular case of impotence, and the greater will be our likelihood of being able to correct the problem.

For a man to experience an erection, his penis needs three things:
• a high-pressure supply of arterial blood
• relaxation of the smooth-muscle tissue
• a functioning blood-storage mechanism to keep blood in the penis and preserve an erection long enough for adequate sexual functioning.

All impotence ultimately results directly from the failure of one of these requirements. And that includes impotence with psychological origins, known as *psychogenic impotence.* Though psychogenic impotence may start "in your head," it ends up affecting what goes on with the penile nerves and blood vessels.

Arteries and Veins

Most parts of the body are connected to the heart by two separate types of blood vessels — *arteries,* which bring fresh blood from the heart and lungs to the body part, and *veins,* which bring "used" blood back from the body part to the heart and lungs where the blood is given fresh oxygen. The arteries, like the water pipes in a house, are under high pressure so that the blood may reach the "upper stories" of the body, such as the brain. The pump that drives this system is the heart itself. The veins, like the drains in a house, are not under high pressure. Blood is able to flow back to the heart and lungs without a strong pump driving it.

Arteries are thick, muscular vessels, which can constrict and maintain the high pressure required. The ability of arteries to expand and constrict allows for control of the amount of blood flowing to an organ at any given time. In this way, blood flow to the muscles of the legs can be increased when you are jogging, and blood flow to the penis can be increased during sexual arousal.

Veins are thin-walled and floppy and are able to expand to drain blood back to the heart as quickly as it is needed.

BLOOD FLOW INTO
AND AWAY FROM THE PENIS

The pathway for blood flow into the penis isn't difficult to understand. If you take a quick glance at the illustration on page 12, you'll notice that cavernosal (erection) arteries run through each corpus cavernosum. These arteries are about 0.6 millimeter in diameter. The blood flowing through them should be at the same pressure as in the arteries of your arm, approximately 120/80 millimeters of mercury.

Blood pressure is normally expressed in millimeters of mercury, written with two numbers in the style of a fraction: The top number is the maximum pressure in the artery, and the bottom number is the minimum pressure. On the other hand, blood pressures from *within the erection chambers* are usually written with one number, also expressed in millimeters of mercury. Pressures *inside the erection chamber* — not the same as within the cavernosal arteries — reflect the maximum arterial pressure during erection minus the pressure lost through blood draining out through the veins during an erection. The normal pressure inside an erection chamber in a patient with an arm blood pressure or a cavernosal artery blood pressure of 120/80 millimeters of mercury is approximately 90 millimeters of mercury— 120 millimeters of maximum arterial pressure minus 30 millimeters of pressure loss through blood draining out through the veins.

Branching off from the cavernosal (erection) arteries are much smaller blood vessels, called *helicine arterioles,* which act as valves controlling arterial blood flow to the erectile tissue (see illustration, page 12).

The arteries going into the two corpora cavernosa function much like an eight-lane highway with many exits. Most of the time, traffic (blood flow) is light—only two lanes are in use and most of the exits are closed.

But during sexual arousal, the vascular equivalent of rush hour takes place. Traffic increases to encompass all eight lanes (the diameter of the arteries almost doubles to 1.2 millimeters), and the muscles around the arterioles relax, allowing high-pressure arterial blood to pump into the lacunar spaces (sinuses) in the corpora cavernosa, initiating an erection.

Veins drain blood away from the penis. During erection, veins inside the corpora cavernosa are squeezed almost (but not completely) shut by the expanded erection tissue pressing against the tunica. When the penis is flaccid, the erection tissue no longer expands against the tunica. The veins inside the corpora cavernosa are open and carry blood outside the tunica and back to the heart.

RELAXATION OF SMOOTH-MUSCLE TISSUE

The body has three types of muscle tissue: *skeletal, cardiac* and *smooth.* Although the conventional view of the penis is that it contains no muscles, what is meant is that it contains no *skeletal* muscles, the type of muscle over which we have voluntary control—like a body builder's muscle. Your penis has none of these—it can't pump iron to make itself bigger.

But it does contain *smooth* muscles. Most of the time we are unaware of our smooth muscles, because they go about their business (with the help of the autonomic nervous system) without our conscious awareness. Smooth muscles contract the walls of our esophagus, stomach and intestines, making digestion possible; they also contract the walls of blood vessels, regulating blood flow. In women, smooth muscles cause the contractions of the uterus, sending the newborn down the birth canal.

In men, smooth-muscle relaxation is crucial to sexual functioning. When smooth muscles in the walls of the tiny blood vessels known as arterioles relax, the supply of blood to the penis is increased. At the same time, relaxation of the smooth-muscle walls

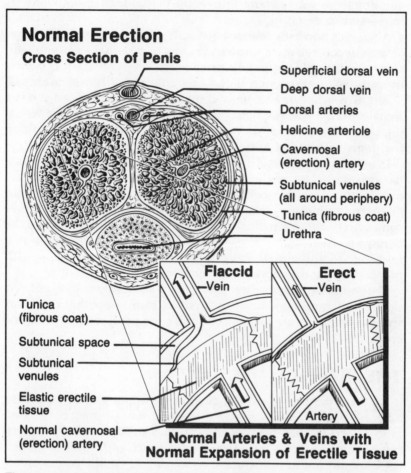

Normal Erection
Cross Section of Penis

- Superficial dorsal vein
- Deep dorsal vein
- Dorsal arteries
- Helicine arteriole
- Cavernosal (erection) artery
- Subtunical venules (all around periphery)
- Tunica (fibrous coat)
- Urethra

Tunica (fibrous coat)

Subtunical space

Subtunical venules

Elastic erectile tissue

Normal cavernosal (erection) artery

Flaccid — Vein

Erect — Vein

Artery

Normal Arteries & Veins with Normal Expansion of Erectile Tissue

The cavernosal artery provides arterial blood to the erection chambers. Subtunical venules drain blood from the lacunar spaces in the periphery of the erection chamber. This venous blood passes into larger veins that enter through the tunica to drain blood away from the penis and ultimately to return it to the heart. In the flaccid state, the smooth muscle of the erection chambers and of the helicine arterioles is constricted, the blood volume and flow into the lacunar spaces is minimal, the subtunical space is open, and the subtunical venules drain freely. In the erect state, the smooth muscle of the erection chambers and of the helicine arterioles is relaxed, the blood volume and flow into the lacunar spaces is maximal, and the subtunical spaces are mechanically compressed by the expanded erection tissue against the fibrous coat, the tunica.

increased. At the same time, relaxation of the smooth-muscle walls in the corpora cavernosa allows the penile lacunar spaces or sinuses to expand during the filling with blood (see illustration, page 13).

Scientists theorize that the interplay between the two parts of the autonomic nervous system controls the behavior of smooth muscles important to erection.

All nerves normally release chemicals called *neurotransmitters*. *Sympathetic* nerves release neurotransmitters that keep the smooth muscles in a state of contraction or constriction—"constricting neurotransmitters"—restricting blood flow into the corpora cavernosa.

But as you become sexually stimulated, the spinal cord sends a signal through *parasympathetic* nerves. These nerves release "relaxing neurotransmitters" that act to *relax* the smooth muscles, flood the penis with blood and help it become erect.

In addition, special cells called *endothelial cells*, which line the lacunar spaces (sinuses) of the corpora cavernosa, may also release chemical agents that either constrict (contract) or relax smooth muscle.

After ejaculation—or after sexual stimulation ceases, whichever comes first—the sympathetic nerves once again take over from the parasympathetic nerves. Constricting neurotransmitters are released into the smooth-muscle cells, blood flow to your penis is again pinched off, and you lose your erection.

Your emotions have a direct effect on your ability to have an erection. If you're upset, worried or anxious, your sympathetic nervous system will dominate the action—and your penis may not become erect.

THE STORAGE MECHANISM

An erect penis holds about eight to ten times as much blood as a flaccid penis. Before arousal, the pressure in your corpora cavernosa (erection chambers) is about 6 to 8 millimeters of mercury, similar to the pressure inside other organs such as the liver or kidney; these organs are low-pressure systems and reflect the *venous* rather than the *arterial* pressure in the body.

Sexual excitement raises the pressure in the corpora cavernosa to that of the arterial system. Blood pressure in the penis zooms upward dramatically—by a factor of ten to fifteen—so that it approximates the high pressure of the body's arteries rather than the low-pressure veins (see box, page 19).

When I perform sophisticated testing on impotent patients, I make sure the overhead TV monitor, which shows pressure in the corpora cavernosa, and the arm blood-pressure monitor, are within the patient's view. As the testing moves along, I invite the patient to watch what happens as his erection (induced by an injection) develops. The tracing representing pressure in the corpora cavernosa moves upward until it approaches the same level as the blood pressure being measured in his arm. Patients usually cheer to encourage the increase in pressure in the penis.

How does the penis accomplish this? The penis is unique among the organs of the body in its ability to *store* blood within itself for a sustained period of time, which is what occurs during sexual stimulation.

As we have seen, the lacunar spaces (sinuses) of the corpora cavernosa swell with blood during periods of sexual excitement, but without a "storage mechanism," nothing would keep the blood in the lacunar spaces. It would be similar to trying to fill a bicycle tire's inner tube that had numerous tiny holes. Just as you started to get up some pressure, the air would rush out the holes. In fact, this approximates what happens with many impotent men (see *Failure to Store*, page 28).

If blood flows into an organ, it must also flow out again, eventually—even in the penis—and that's where the penile veins come in. In the illustration on page 21, you'll see the arteries buried deep inside the corpora cavernosa; in contrast, the *veins* (actually, the subtunical venules) of the corpora cavernosa lie practically on its surface. Arteries carry blood from the heart to an organ; veins carry it back to the heart. The veins of the penis drain blood away from the erectile tissue back to the heart.

As we shall see, the fact that venous (vein) blood leaves the penis's erectile tissue *close to its surface* is critical for the penis's storage mechanism.

A net of specialized veins called *subtunical venules* (venules are "little veins"—here approximately 0.1 millimeter in size) drains blood from the peripheral lacunar spaces (sinuses). The blood feeds into larger and larger tributaries, *emissary veins*, until it reaches either of the principal veins of the penis running into the pelvis.

Remember: *Blood enters the corpora cavernosa from deep inside their centers; blood leaves the corpora from their surfaces.*

The *tunica albuginea* surrounds each corpus cavernosum (that's the singular for corpora cavernosa). If you think of the tunica as a hard rubber tire enclosing a soft inner tube of erection tissue, you can begin to understand the storage mechanism.

The subtunical venules behave like tiny leaks in the inner tube. They let blood that is flowing into the penis leak back out again—which is fine, except when you want to have an erection. Ordinarily, when you pump air into a leaky bicycle tire, most of the air escapes into the space between the inner tube and the walls of the tire.

But suppose you pump ten times as fast as normal—and the tube is able to expand despite the leaks. Where the surface of the expanding tube meets the wall, air can no longer escape. As you continue furiously pumping, less and less air leaks, and the tube expands faster and faster. Eventually, the pressure of the tube against the tire wall closes all the leaks.

A similar process occurs with an erection. As the lacunar spaces fill with blood during erection, they expand; the engorged lacunar spaces press the subtunical venules against the tunica. At a certain point, the venules are pressed flat. Only a trickle of blood escapes through the veins. The corpora cavernosa swell to their full capacity and maintain the full erection of the penis (illustration, page 21).

In the section *Failure to Store* (page 28), we will discuss what can go wrong with the storage mechanism.

The Potency Spectrum

A patient of mine who was an avid reader once mentioned an illustration he'd seen in a popular men's magazine. A series of translucent erections, each less rigid (pointing further toward the ground) than the next, had been superimposed atop one another on a man's torso. Each of the erections had been labeled—"16 years old," "30 years old," "50 years old" and "70 years old." My patient wanted to know how aging influenced erections, even, as the illustration suggested, among healthy men.

Theoretically, an older man's erections should not be inferior in quality to those of a younger man. However, the time it takes for the penis to "recover" after an orgasm and become erect again (known as the "refractory period"), and the time from initial arousal to orgasm are both longer in an older man.

And, we can show statistically that the erections of many men—perhaps *most* men—will decline as a result of *organic damage* to the penis. This means that for a host of reasons, including lifestyle, aging, genetic predisposition and pelvic injury, most men will experience some decline either in the flow of blood into the penis, in the ability of their erectile smooth-muscle tissue to relax adequately or in their blood-storage mechanism.

The key to recognizing that you have a problem is watching for consistent change in your established pattern of erections. The vast majority of men who complain of problems do not become impotent overnight, nor are they impotent in all circumstances.

The distinctions outlined below regarding the quality of erections apply to the ability of the penis to become erect in three situations—when having intercourse, when masturbating and when sleeping (the average man has four erections per night while sleeping).

Erectile Potency. Generally, potency is taken to mean having erections that are sufficiently rigid to achieve penetration during intercourse, and being able to maintain an erection until ejaculation—most of the time. But even for a man with normal erectile potency, there are times when stress, anxiety or simple fatigue get the best of his erections. It is also possible for a man to have some minimal organic

How Age Affects Erections

Many studies, including data from the famous sex researcher Alfred Kinsey, suggest that approximately 10 percent of men are impotent by age fifty, with a virtual doubling of that percentage for each of the following decades: 20 percent at age sixty, 40 percent at age seventy and 80 percent at age eighty. Under age 30, the incidence of impotence is less than 2 percent.

There is very little about aging that is very good for an erection. The ravages of disease, surgery, medication and the vascular risk factors mentioned in chapter 1 — high blood pressure, cigarette smoking, diabetes and high cholesterol — may all adversely influence overall erectile performance.

The testicles make less testosterone. Sensory nerves become less receptive. The amount of neurotransmitter released by the nerves that control smooth-muscle tissue declines as we age. Atherosclerosis catches up with arteries, reducing the pressure available to achieve rigidity in an erection. The erectile tissue itself undergoes biochemical reactions that cause it to stiffen and become less elastic; these changes affect the storage mechanism.

There are psychological hurdles, too. The aging man has to combat the attitude that he is too old to have sex, that sex is only for young people and that he has already had his fling.

Still, there's no reason why a man can't remain sexually active for as long as he wants. The important news is that if a man wishes to maintain his erections, he may be able to prevent many of the problems of aging by keeping his blood pressure under control, watching his blood cholesterol and exercising regularly. If problems do develop, he can undergo an evaluation and choose from a variety of treatment options.

damage that interferes with a normal physiologic erection and still be able to become sufficiently erect for intercourse and to achieve orgasm.

Normal Physiologic Erections. These are erections in which the blood pressure in the corpora cavernosa approximates the blood pressure in the your arm. These erections are quite hard — usually about 90 millimeters of mercury — and last easily more than ten minutes.

Erectile Insufficiency. An insufficiency describes a consistent change in erections in all three circumstances — during intercourse, during masturbation and during sleep. This change may be in how rigid your penis becomes or how long your erection lasts. Since almost every man has suffered an occasional instance of poor erections, the key to diagnosing an insufficiency is noticing a consistent, distinct *difference over time,* usually for at least a year. Men with an insufficiency are by far the largest group of patients seeking help with their potency. They are usually potent some of the time. We have found that over 90 percent of men with erectile insufficiency have some sort of vascular (blood-vessel) damage — either a blockage in the artery to the penis, or erectile tissue that's too stiff to expand easily against the tunica to enable adequate storage of blood.

Erectile Failure. This term implies the consistent inability for at least a year in any of the three situations — during intercourse, masturbation or sleep — to achieve an erection sufficient for penetration or to sustain penetration until ejaculation. Men with erectile failure are rarely potent, and organic damage to the mechanisms of erection is virtually always at the root of the problem.

Initiating, Filling and Storing — the Erection Problem Areas

If your penis isn't getting enough blood, or if your smooth-muscle tissue either won't or can't relax, then you're going to have problems with your erections.

What follows is a summary of the three problem areas of erectile performance — difficulties in "initiating," "filling" and "storing" (see illustrations, pages 29 and 30).

FAILURE TO INITIATE

"Failure to initiate" is a fancy way of describing what happens when important nerves in the penis fail to function correctly in response to sexual stimulation. As a consequence, arteries in the penis do not dilate properly and the lacunar spaces in the penis's erectile tissue remain contracted, unable to absorb blood and expand. In a word, everything stays squeezed shut, and the process of erection cannot begin.

Spinal-cord injuries, multiple sclerosis and radical pelvic surgery are frequent causes of this type of nerve malfunction. Nerve-damaging pelvic fractures can also cause the penis to fail to initiate. Also, many patients with *diabetes mellitus* fail to initiate, but they often have vascular problems as well. (See chapter 8 for a more complete discussion of the problems of men with neurologic problems and diabetes mellitus.)

Low hormone levels may on occasion be the cause of a "failure to initiate" because hormones are necessary for sexual desire to occur.

The mind-body connection is also apparent with the problem of failure to initiate. The spinal reflex centers that control erection are also connected to higher centers in the brain. Anxious thoughts, stress, worries — all of these have an influence on the signals being transmitted from your spinal cord to your penis. If your emotional state causes your sympathetic nervous system to predominate, then your penile tissues — smooth-muscle tissue in both the arteries and the lacunar spaces — receive more signals to contract than to relax, and your penis doesn't get enough blood to become erect.

FAILURE TO FILL

"Failure to fill" means just that — not enough arterial, high-pressure blood gets to the penis to expand the erectile tissue. Typically, this occurs as the result of a difference in the blood pressure in the *cavernosal arteries* — the arteries that supply blood to the corpora cavernosa — from the blood pressure in the arteries of the rest of the body. The medical phrase is "cavernosal artery insufficiency." During sexual stimulation, arterial blood should enter the penis at a dramatically increased rate. When a patient has a problem "filling," the blood pressure in his arteries is not high enough to greatly increase the pressure in the erectile tissue, usually because of an obstruction somewhere in the arteries to the penis (see illustration, page 29).

Blockages may be either localized in one or two spots or widely distributed throughout the pelvic arterial system or even involve the arteries within the penis.

Localized blockages tend to be associated with accidental injuries to the *perineum* (the area between the anus and the scrotum), often the result of a fall or blow to that area, although the effect of the injury ("trauma" in medical language) may not show up for years. There may be no problem with erectile functioning until additional deterioration in blood flow, initiated by the trauma, begins to interfere with filling.

I've had patients recollect long-ago falls on basketball courts, falls on fences and on protruding objects, motorcycle accidents, damaging bicycle rides, even beatings in World War II prison camps, when I point out that a blow or shock to the part of the penis hidden beneath the perineum can precipitate arterial blockages, and therefore impotence.

The second type of blockages, the ones that are diffuse throughout the pelvic arterial system, are often the result of *atherosclerosis* (harden-ing and narrowing of the arteries).

Cigarette smoking, hypertension, a high cholesterol level, diabetes mellitus, X-ray treatments, stress and a family history of vascular disease are all associated with this condition. Some of these risk fac-tors are beyond your control, but two of the most influential ones— smoking and diet—are not.

If you're still smoking—stop. If you don't know how much fat your diet contains, refer to the last chapter of this book to find out how to eat properly, and have your blood cholesterol level tested regularly.

FAILURE TO STORE

For an erection's storage mechanism to function properly, you need proper relaxation of the penis's smooth-muscle tissue (in the walls of the penile arteries and in the walls of the lacunar spaces) and elasticity of the erectile tissue. The penis has to store blood to re-main erect.

If you pump hard enough, you may be able to inflate a leaky tire, but as soon as your effort slackens, the tire will deflate. So, even with an adequate flow of arterial blood into the penis, a leaky storage system will prevent a lasting, firm erection.

Veins will continue to drain blood out of the corpora cavernosa (erection chambers) when for some reason the muscles of the penis fail to relax, or the the tissues of the corpora cavernosa fail to ex-pand sufficiently to press up against the veins and compress them and pinch them shut.

This may mean that the smooth-muscle tissue is not getting the correct signals from the nervous system or enough of the chemical relaxants from the cells of the lacunar spaces (see illustration, page 13)—or it may simply indicate that the erectile tissue itself has lost its elasticity.

Right now, we think that the loss of elasticity in these erectile tissues results from the scarring or stiffening caused by the same condi-tions that damage the walls of arteries—smoking, high cholesterol, hypertension, diabetes mellitus, injury and aging.

In animal experiments, we've been able to study a possible rela-tionship between hardening of the arteries, high cholesterol and the effectiveness of the animals' storage mechanisms during the erec-tion process. The results from animal experimentation require more investigation, but thus far they seem to bear out our conclusions regarding the impotent men with "storage" problems that we see in our clinic.

Artery Blockage Causing 'Failure to Fill'

Cross Section of Penis

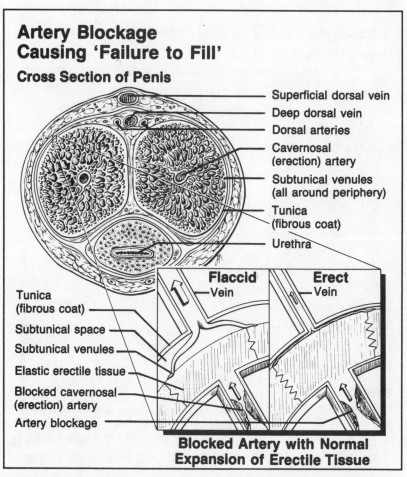

Superficial dorsal vein

Deep dorsal vein

Dorsal arteries

Cavernosal (erection) artery

Subtunical venules (all around periphery)

Tunica (fibrous coat)

Urethra

Tunica (fibrous coat)

Subtunical space

Subtunical venules

Elastic erectile tissue

Blocked cavernosal (erection) artery

Artery blockage

Flaccid Vein

Erect Vein

Blocked Artery with Normal Expansion of Erectile Tissue

In "failure-to-fill" erection insufficiency, the cavernosal or erection artery has blockages that lower the pressure and the flow of blood reaching the erection chamber, adversely affecting erections. Blockages may be the result of blunt trauma to the artery, or more commonly, of hardening of the arteries or atherosclerosis. With failure to fill, erections develop more slowly than is normal, though they may eventually become sufficiently rigid for intercourse.

Leakage from Veins ('Failure to Store')

Cross Section of Penis

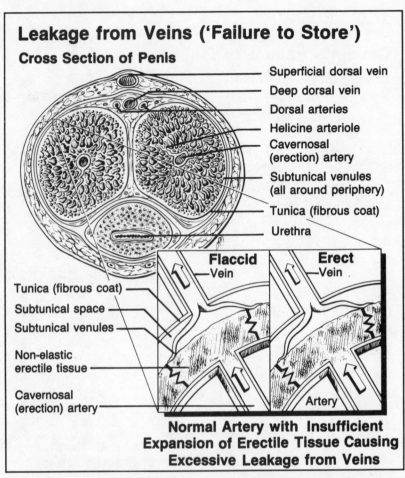

Superficial dorsal vein

Deep dorsal vein

Dorsal arteries

Helicine arteriole

Cavernosal (erection) artery

Subtunical venules (all around periphery)

Tunica (fibrous coat)

Urethra

Tunica (fibrous coat)

Subtunical space

Subtunical venules

Non-elastic erectile tissue

Cavernosal (erection) artery

Flaccid —Vein

Erect —Vein

Artery

Normal Artery with Insufficient Expansion of Erectile Tissue Causing Excessive Leakage from Veins

In "failure-to-store" erection insufficiency, the erection tissue is unable to maximally expand during erection against the fibrous coat, the tunica. The subtunical space remains open, and the subtunical venules drain freely, allowing blood to escape during erection. The erection tissue cannot expand adequately if the smooth-muscle tissue within it remains contracted from anxiety or if the erection tissue is stiff from scarring or if changes in the quality of the erection tissue have occurred from aging or vascular disease. With failure to store, erections are difficult to sustain and are usually not rigid enough for intercourse.

Treatment Options for Erection Problems

The treatment options available for the patient with erection problems include:

- **Psychological (Sex) Therapy**
- **Oral, Topical and Intramuscular Medications**
- **Vacuum Constriction Devices**
- **Self-Injection Therapy**
- **Vascular Surgery for Artery Blockages**
- **Vascular Surgery for Storage Problems**
- **Penile Implant Surgery**

I have arranged them from the most conservative, reversible, noninvasive treatment option to the most invasive, irreversible treatment option. To help with your understanding of these various treatments, each one is summarized in a brief explanation of the treatment, the indications for it and by the advantages and disadvantages of the treatment.

SEX THERAPY AND OTHER COUNSELING

The goal of modern, behaviorally oriented sex therapy and counseling is to restore potency by focusing on such problems as excessive anxiety, sexual inhibition or communication problems between sex partners. One aspect of this treatment is *sensate focus exercises*, which are designed to progressively and slowly improve erection performance by showing couples how to enjoy non-intercourse sexual activity. Couples are usually treated as a unit from as few as six sessions to as many as fifteen to thirty sessions with sessions decreasing in frequency over time. Sex therapy is discussed in detail in chapter 3.

When Is Sex Therapy or Counseling Indicated?

Sex therapy or counseling is indicated both for the patient with psychogenic impotence (without physical factors) as well as for the patient with physical factors causing impotence who is also experiencing psychological or relationship problems.

Advantages

Sex therapy is reversible, does not involve the use of oral or injectable medication and does not require surgery with its associated requirements of anesthesia, wound healing and recovery time away from work. Psychological reactions to erection problems, even if the problems are physical, are extremely common and may adversely influence the success of any of the physical treatments for impotence. Sex therapy therefore has wide applicability in the treatment of problems with erections. Sex therapy and related forms of counseling do not involve an extremely long time commitment compared to more formal psychotherapy. Short-term sex therapy commonly lasts approximately fifteen weeks.

Disadvantages

The reported success rates with psychological therapy have varied widely, from 35 to 80 percent in different studies. Follow-up studies on people who have had sex therapy suggest that there is a significant recurrence of impotence with time after sex therapy treatment, especially in patients with long-term erection problems who are older or have diminished sexual interest. A physical exam and evaluation by a urologist should precede a commitment to sex therapy.

ORAL, TOPICAL AND INTRAMUSCULAR MEDICATIONS

The goal of these medications is to restore potency and sex drive in impotent patients by providing them with treatment that is directed at a specific physical abnormality that is causing the erection problem.

The most successful medical therapy for the impotent patient has been the treatment of hormonal problems that cause a decreased level of sexual desire and "failure to initiate" (see page 26). The aim of hormonal therapy for impotent patients is to maintain normal levels of hormones. Treatment with testosterone, given in intramuscular injections, is the most common form of hormonal therapy. See *Low Testosterone and Other Hormonal Disorders,* page 157.

Other drug therapies that have been proposed, but are still experimental, include use of oral agents to dilate arteries, to block the harmful effects of adrenaline, to increase zinc levels and to act as aphrodisiacs. Skin pastes to dilate arteries and relax smooth-muscle tissues are also in the experimental stage at this time.

When Are These Medications Indicated?

Hormonal treatment is indicated only in patients with abnormal levels of hormones who are having erectile problems. In the past, testosterone has been over-prescribed for erectile problems not related to hormonal deficiencies.

Treatment with oral medications or skin pastes may be desired for treatment of failure-to-initiate, failure-to-fill or failure-to-store erection problems, but as yet there are no oral medications or skin pastes that are recognized with statistical proof to be effective for the treatment of organic impotence.

Advantages

Treatment with testosterone, which is usually injected into the muscles around the buttocks, is more comfortable, less invasive and less risky than injection of drugs into the penis itself or surgery on the penile structures. It is also an advantage in that it is a specific corrective treatment for patients who are deficient in testosterone, restoring normal levels of this hormone.

Disadvantages

In patients requiring replacement of testosterone because of low levels of testosterone, oral medication has been found to be less effective and has been associated with side effects of liver damage and abnormal blood fat levels. Intramuscular injections are preferable, but should be given approximately every three weeks, which can be inconvenient and uncomfortable.

In addition, many impotent men are in the older age group and thus in the age group found to have the highest prevalence of cancer of the prostate. Use of testosterone in such patients may possibly encourage the growth of prostate cancer if a cancer is already present but undetected.

VACUUM CONSTRICTION DEVICES

The goal of *vacuum constrictive devices* (VCDs) is to restore potency by creating a vacuum-generated negative pressure around the penile shaft, which enables blood to accumulate in the penile shaft. A constriction band is placed at the base of the penis to maintain the penile shaft erection. See box, page 169 and the illustration on page 170 for more information about VCDs.

When Is the Vacuum Constriction Device Indicated?

This treatment is indicated in patients who have been found by testing to have erection problems as a result of physical factors such as failure to initiate, fill or store and who do not desire or are not good candidates for surgery or other treatments. The VCD may also be utilized in patients with psychogenic impotence where counseling and sex therapy are not desired or have not been effective.

Advantages

Vacuum constrictive devices are external devices in that they are placed over the skin of the penis. They do not require surgery with its associated requirements of anesthesia, wound healing and recovery time away from work, and they do not require the patient to inject himself.

Disadvantages

Complications of this therapy include: difficulties with ejaculation in view of the elastic band placed around the penis blocking the urethra; and penile pain, penile bruising or foreskin swelling from excessive negative pressure applied to the penile skin. This treatment option has apparently been utilized by some impotent patients for several years but only recently has become a popular and accepted treatment alternative. There are therefore very few published prospective studies on its long-term safety, efficacy and patient acceptance in the treatment of impotence.

SELF-INJECTION THERAPY

The goal of self-injection therapy is to restore potency by injecting drugs into the erection chambers that relax the smooth-muscle tissues of the penis and allow erection to take place. See chapter 6 for a complete discussion of self-injection therapy and the medications that are used in the injections.

When Is Self-Injection Therapy Indicated?

This treatment is indicated in patients who have been found by testing to have physical erection problems as a result of nerve damage (failure to initiate), artery blockages (failure to fill) or storage problems (failure to store). Patients with psychogenic impotence can also be candidates for self-injection therapy, especially if the erection problem is not restored by the more standard treatment of psychological or sex therapy.

Advantages

Self-injection therapy attempts to mimic the natural physical mechanisms that occur following sexual stimulation — that is, relaxation of the smooth-muscle tissues of the penis. Functional erections usually result in a variable time — ten to thirty minutes — following the injection. Penile injections are dependable and have had widespread patient acceptance. This treatment option enables restoration of erections without the need for surgery and its associated requirements of anesthesia, wound healing and recovery time away from work. The injections do not influence penile sensation, ejaculation or fertility, nor do they affect the patient's partner.

Disadvantages

Self-injection requires the training of self-injection techniques that can be performed by the patient in his home. Patients must undergo a dosage determination in which the lowest possible dose is identified that results in an erection.

Patients who have poor manual dexterity, poor vision or severe obesity may not be appropriate candidates for self-injection therapy. The medications in the injections may pose a problem for patients who also have heart disease, previous strokes or blood disorders.

Complications of treatment include rare infection, pain and burning and the problem of prolonged erections. Prolonged erections occur in approximately 2 to 15 percent of injection users, most often during the period when their correct dosage is being determined. The problem occurs in less than 1 percent of injection users once their correct dosage has been determined. Since prolonged erections can damage the penile tissues, patients are cautioned to report to their doctor any erection that lasts longer than four hours.

Other rare complications include fainting and a remote possibility of liver injury. Long-term side effects of penile injection therapy are unknown because the treatment has only been available since 1983.

REVASCULARIZATION (BYPASS) SURGERY FOR ARTERY BLOCKAGES

The goal of *revascularization* surgery (also called bypass surgery) for artery blockages is to restore potency by increasing blood flow to the penis by bypassing artery blockages. For more information about revascularization (bypass) procedures, see chapter 4 and the illustration on page 82.

When Is Revascularization Surgery Indicated?

This procedure is indicated in patients who have been found by testing to have erection problems as a result of artery blockages and whose artery blockages are able to be effectively bypassed. Since erections depend not only on the flow of blood into the erection chamber but on how effectively the blood is stored in the erection chambers during erection, it is important to have both these mechanisms evaluated before undergoing treatment for artery blockages.

Advantages

Restoration of potency by vascular surgery in appropriate cases enables the patient's own natural erection to be used without further treatments.

Disadvantages

The results of vascular surgery for artery blockages to restore erections have varied from a 31 percent to an 80 percent success rate in different studies. Younger men who have few areas of blockages in their arteries generally do better than older men and those who have more widespread (diffuse) areas of blockage, which are difficult to bypass. Surgery generally is prolonged, often lasting four to eight hours. A recovery period lasting six weeks is advised before resuming both strenuous physical as well as sexual activity. Complications with surgery are rare but do occur and may include infection, pain and disruption of the bypass, especially if sexual activity is resumed before healing is complete.

VASCULAR SURGERY FOR STORAGE PROBLEMS

Vascular surgery for storage problems involves tying off or actually removing the veins that are causing excessive drainage of blood away from the erection chambers or tightening the tunica that surrounds the erection chambers so that its compression of the penile veins is more easily accomplished. These procedures are known as *venous ligation* and *crural plication*, respectively. They both restore potency by decreasing excessive drainage of blood from the erection chambers during erection. For more information about these procedures, see chapter 5 and the illustrations on pages 104 and 107.

When Is Vascular Surgery for Storage Problems Indicated?

These surgical procedures are indicated in patients who have been found by testing to have erection problems as a result of storage problems. Since erections depend not only how effectively blood is stored in the erection chambers during erection but also on the flow of blood entering into the erection chamber, it is important to have both mechanisms evaluated before undergoing treatment for storage problems.

Advantages

Restoration of potency by vascular surgery in appropriate cases enables the patient's own natural erection to be used without further treatments.

Disadvantages

The success rate of vascular surgery for storage problems in restoring erections ranges from 28 percent to 73 percent in different studies. Patients who are younger, have few areas of storage abnormalities and whose areas of excessive drainage are able to be reduced by surgery have predictably more success in restoring functional erections than patients who are older, have more widespread areas of storage problems and whose areas of excessive drainage are not able to be effectively diminished by surgery. Surgery generally lasts two to three hours, but may be longer. A recovery period lasting four to six weeks is advised before resuming both strenuous physical as well as sexual activity. Complications with surgery may include infection, pain, shortening of the penis and numbness of the penis.

PENILE IMPLANT SURGERY

The goal of penile implant surgery is to restore potency by surgically implanting a mechanical device known as an *implant* into the erection chambers that provides penile rigidity sufficient for intercourse. For details about penile implants, see chapter 7 and the illustrations on pages 134 and 136.

When Is Penile Implant Surgery Indicated?

This procedure is indicated in patients who have been found by testing to have erection problems as a result of physical factors such as failure to initiate, failure to fill or failure to store and who are not good candidates for vascular surgery to restore their own erections because, for example, their vascular or tissue damage is too widespread. Penile implants are sometimes recommended for patients with psychogenic impotence if psychotherapy or other treatments have not been successful or are not desired.

Advantages

The postoperative satisfaction rate for implant surgery from the standpoint of the patient and his sexual partner has been reported to be approximately 90 percent. This makes treatment by penile implant one of the most successful of all treatment options for patients with impotence. This treatment option has been available since the early 1970s, so there is much data available on usage, success rates and complications. Approximately twenty-five thousand penile implant devices are implanted in the United States each year. Penile sensation as well as the ability to ejaculate and reach orgasm are usually not changed by a penile implant.

Disadvantages

Treatment by penile implant is irreversible in that insertion of the implant device into the erection chambers permanently injures the erection tissue. For this reason, treatment with the penile implant is generally utilized as a *last* treatment option.

Surgery generally lasts one to two hours but may be longer depending on the type of implant chosen. A recovery period lasting four to six weeks is advised before resuming both strenuous physical as well as sexual activity. Postoperative pain can be expected to require narcotic pain relief and last up to four weeks.

Complications have been reported with the penile implants, including: infection of the device in approximately 1 to 8 percent of cases; movement of the device from the erection chamber to the skin or to another body part (such as the urethra) in approximately 1 percent of cases; and mechanical failure of the device or connecting tubes in approximately 2 to 10 percent of cases. When such complications do occur, the implant device is usually removed and a new implant device is inserted during the same or during another operative procedure. The quality of the patient's original normal erections in terms of penile size, length and hardness will not be exactly restored by the penile implant. In most cases the implant erection will not be as long and not be as wide as before the impotence.

SUMMARY OF SYMPTOMS, CAUSES AND TREATMENTS OF IMPOTENCE

TYPE OF IMPOTENCE	SYMPTOMS*	CAUSES	TREATMENTS
Failure to Initiate	Inability to initiate (develop) an erection.	Nerve damage due to disease or injury; stress, anxiety or other psychological problems; hormonal disorders.	Sex therapy, hormonal therapy, vacuum constriction device, penile injections, penile implant.
Failure to Fill**	Erections develop slowly and may not be sufficiently rigid for intercourse or masturbation except sometimes after extended foreplay or stimulation; sleep erections or erections upon awakening may appear more rigid.	Arterial blockage(s) due to atherosclerosis, aging or injury.	Sex therapy, vacuum constriction device, revascularization surgery (arterial bypass surgery), penile implant.
Failure to Store**	Erections poorly maintained and not rigid enough for intercourse or masturbation.	Abnormal storage due to stress, aging, injury or any process that causes erectile tissue to stiffen and not expand enough to compress subtunical venules.	Sex therapy, vacuum constriction device, penile injections, venous ligation surgery, crural plication surgery, penile implant.

*Changes in erections (in rigidity or sustaining capability or both) must occur with morning erections, during masturbation and during intercourse for a period of six months to a year before the patient is considered in need of treatment for impotence.

**Failure-to-fill impotence and failure-to-store impotence often occur together as the result of a disease process, atherosclerosis or aging.

Impotence Prevention

Before we go on to the case histories of some of my patients, I'd like to emphasize that there is hope that prevention of some kinds of potency problems may be possible with diet, exercise and other behavioral changes.

We have little influence over the accidents that befall us in life, and even less over our genetic makeup. But vital decisions about what we eat, whether we exercise and whether or not we smoke, may have a direct effect on the quality of our erections.

Hardly a month goes by without a new revelation reaching the popular press concerning the influence of diet and smoking on vascular disease. Atherosclerosis results when various deposits cling to arterial walls. As this fatty sludge builds up, the space for blood flow becomes progressively smaller; the body's blood pressure increases, causing further arterial damage. Scar tissue in the arterial walls and increased blockage are the net result, both of which make the blood vessels stiffer, less able to stretch and recover their shape.

It stands to reason that the penis, as one of the most vascular organs in the human body, would suffer greatly from those things that impair the ability of blood-vessel tissues to stretch and recover their shape. As a rule of thumb, what's good for your heart and legs is good for your erections; what's bad for your heart and legs may be *worse* for your penis.

———— ♦ ————

In the next chapter you'll read more about the mind-body connection in impotence and you'll learn about the role of sex therapy in impotence treatment. Although I've emphasized so far that most impotence is caused primarily by physical factors, that doesn't mean that psychological factors are not also involved; and, for most men, physiologically based impotence causes a great deal of anxiety, frustration and psychic pain. Sex therapists and other kinds of counselors can help impotent men and their partners overcome the psychological blocks to their potency, whether or not psychological factors are the main cause of the problem.

CHAPTER 3

The Mind-Body Connection and the Role of Sex Therapy

by Dr. Alma Dell Smith

Dr. Alma Dell Smith is the author of this chapter. She is a psychologist who specializes in sex therapy, and for many years I have relied on her insight into the psychological aspects of impotence, often referring patients to her practice for treatment. She contributed this chapter as well as comments on several of the patients presented in subsequent chapters. Dr. Smith saw Jim and Mary Campbell, whose story is told at the end of this chapter, as sex therapy patients. She evaluated the surgical patients described elsewhere in this book either in person or by studying their histories and interviews. The names and biographical details for all patients in this book have been changed, although the medical facts have not. The patients described graciously allowed me to include their case histories and allowed Dr. Smith to review and comment on them as well.
— Irwin Goldstein, M.D.

Psychogenic Impotence

Until very recently, almost all impotence was attributed to psychological causes. That's why this book took so much time in chapter 2 to explain the physiology of erectile functioning and to reassure you that impotence is *not* usually "all in your head." On the other hand, organic impotence *may* also involve psychological factors. That's where psychologists and sex therapists come into the treatment picture.

If you're experiencing problems with your erections, the first thing you ought to do—besides reading this book—is make an appointment with a physician who specializes in impotence evaluation and treatment. Usually, this will be a urologist.

The urologist will attempt to separate the physical and psychological components. Urologists diagnose and treat the physical aspects of impotence; psychologists and sex therapists address the psychological side of the problem.

Sometimes, a urologist will recommend sex therapy even if the psychological factors are secondary to the physical ones. In these cases, sex therapists can help determine your suitability for certain surgical procedures, such as a penile implant, or help you with the emotional adjustment after vascular reconstructive surgery or other treatment for impotence. They can also prevent a physical problem from being a bigger impediment to a man's sex life than it has to be.

But the urologist will most often recommend sex therapy if he or she believes your problem is predominantly psychological. Urologists don't make such a determination lightly. Little or no damage to your erectile physiology, rigid, well-sustained nocturnal (nighttime—while sleeping) erections, normal erections during masturbation or fantasizing, normal hormone levels, functioning nerves, adequate blood flow and effective blood storage—all of these may point to *psychogenic*, or psychologically caused, impotence as opposed to *organic*, or physiologically caused, impotence.

This doesn't mean that psychogenic impotence is any less "real" than organic impotence. The man with psychogenic impotence has a very real problem—he's just as impotent as a man with a physical problem. His penis fails to become erect for very sound reasons. But, unlike a man with organic impotence, his problem *starts in his mind*, not in damage or impairment to his body. Men with psychogenic impotence inadvertently sabotage their own erections through disruptive thoughts, worries and self-judgments. Their anxious state causes the release of adrenaline-like chemicals (neurotransmitters) that constrict the smooth-muscle tissue of the penis and its arteries, reducing blood inflow from the arteries and increasing blood outflow away from the penis. The end result is flaccidity rather than erection (see *Failure to Initiate*, pages 26 and 27 and illustration, page 13).

If the urologist concludes that a man's problem is primarily psychological—and if the patient seems receptive to examining some of his ideas and patterns of sexual behavior—he should be referred to a counselor, usually a sex therapist. Sex therapy may be effective in restoring potency, especially if both partners of a couple become involved in the treatment.

THE MIND-BODY CONNECTION

The mind is a hidden, but influential, part of our sexual makeup. Most men never consider their sexual psychology until something goes wrong, and self-doubt begins filling their heads.

For example, a man who has just started taking medication for hypertension may try making love to his partner one night, when suddenly and quite puzzlingly, he finds himself losing his erection. Nothing like this has ever happened to him before. He tries not to worry about it. Several nights later the same thing occurs—and this time his mind races with panic: What's wrong with me? Am I losing my desire for my partner? The woman, perhaps sympathetic but unsure how to react, says nothing. He immediately assumes the worst—that she's judging him and finding him inadequate.

Almost certainly, the next time they make love he'll have to wrestle with anxiety, distracting him from his lovemaking, and initiating a vicious cycle of failure leading to anxiety leading to more failure, and so on. The root cause of this man's problem may be primarily physical, a byproduct of his blood-pressure medication (see *Medication-Associated Impotence,* page 171), but it soon acquires a secondary psychological dimension. His internist may adjust his blood-pressure medication, but unless the couple addresses the psychological aspects of the problem, they may be in for more difficulty in the future.

Likewise, a man may have only a small amount of vascular damage in his penis, so little that it seemingly doesn't impair his erections at all. But then comes a day when a new boss, a real fire breather, replaces his old superior. Double your sales in ninety days, the new boss demands, or start looking for a new job. That night the man fails to become erect when he tries to make love. Things only get worse over the course of the next week as his wife assures him that his erections aren't that important to her. They're not, eh? Well, they're damn important to me!

A urological workup subsequently reveals a minor blood-storage abnormality in the man's erections, but not enough to warrant drug treatment or surgery. At the urologist's suggestion the man has an interview with a psychologist. The interview reveals the depth of the impotent man's anxiety over his job security and his high stress level.

At this point, he has several non-surgical options: He can correct his vascular problem by availing himself of an injection program he learned about in the urologist's office (see chapter 6); he and his partner can participate in short-term sex therapy, where they will learn to improve their sexual communication so that the man's job pressure doesn't hold their love life hostage; or he may combine the two, perhaps utilizing the injection therapy for a brief period while he learns to diminish his anxiety.

Sex therapy offers benefits for men suffering from all types of impotence *as long as appropriate measures are taken simultaneously to treat whatever organic problems may also be present.*

Erectile difficulties that last for several months or more, regardless of their cause, inevitably disrupt a couple's relationship. Correcting the physical problem does not necessarily restore the original harmony, and that's another role for sex therapy—to help the couple recover from the trauma that impotence has inflicted on their love life.

Successful Sex

Chapter 2 emphasized physiology—it identified the parts of the male reproductive system and explained how those parts collaborate to cause an erection. But successful sexual functioning also requires the participation of certain other factors which, while less tangible than physical things, are just as important. Our experiences, attitudes, emotions and relationships create a mental framework that either enhances or sabotages successful sexual functioning. In addition to adequate physiology (*adequate,* by the way, not *perfect*), a man needs three things:

• the right sexual stimulation (both physical and emotional)
• a history of positive sexual experiences
• the absence of severe stress symptoms, distracting thoughts or feelings of depression.

THE RIGHT STIMULATION

"Right stimulation" means satisfying a man's particular sexual tastes. It may involve any of the five senses, by themselves or in combination with a thousand different fantasies. Perspiration, perfume and vaginal aroma may be strongly stimulating to one man and not another, or they may be more or less stimulating to the same man depending on the time of day or physical surroundings. What is exciting on the third day of a vacation with an empty afternoon stretching languorously ahead of you may not produce the same effect the night before an important business trip.

What a man finds stimulating may in part depend on memories of early experiences or early masturbation fantasies. A man may find himself with strong preferences in body shape—for example, slim hips and large breasts, and he may not find the body of a woman with small breasts or large hips as inherently arousing.

A large part of "what turns you on" is highly personal, but a lot of it is also connected with social conditioning. A survey of the history of "desirable" female shapes shows an astonishing variability from era to era, and lately, even from decade to decade. The aerobicized athleticism of Bo Derek and Grace Jones, reflecting our current obsession with physical fitness, would seem startlingly unappealing only a generation ago when the voluptuous sexiness of Marilyn Monroe and Sophia Loren held sway.

Few of us are perfect, however, no matter what the current standards are.

If the visual stimulation provided by his partner is not "perfect," a man may want to focus on her skin texture or their love feelings, directing his attention to his partner's appealing attributes, rather than the negative ones.

If a man is being insufficiently stimulated by his partner because she does not match his idea of a sexually stimulating woman, and if he cannot get past that, he may be more prone to the adverse influences of organic factors such as impaired artery inflow or abnormal blood storage.

———— ♦ ————

As a man grows older, more and more direct stimulation to his penis may be necessary to accomplish what simple thought or fantasy would have done in his younger years. Couples need to understand this and take it into account in their sexual style.

For young men, problems with sustaining an erection or with ejaculation may be related to the differences between the physical sensations of masturbation and the somewhat different feelings of vaginal stimulation in intercourse. They too may need education and adjustment to have satisfying sexual relations.

COMMUNICATION SKILLS TO IMPROVE STIMULATION

Sex therapists try to treat couples suffering from problems of insufficient or inappropriate stimulation by improving partners' communication skills.

One way that sex therapists have of improving those skills is through the teaching of *sensate focus* exercises. Sensate focus exercises, developed by Dr. William Masters and Dr. Virginia Johnson in the late 1960s, teach couples how to caress each other and communicate with each other physically, at first without having intercourse or reaching orgasm. By learning how to express their sexual likes and dislikes in this way, couples add a spirit of flexibility into their lovemaking, adjusting their mutual stimulation toward what most excites them.

POSITIVE SEXUAL EXPERIENCES

Cultural messages, family attitudes and partner reactions can all contribute to your attitude toward sexuality. Religious teachings, books, peer pressure and early sexual experiences all bring their influence to bear. The quality of early sexual impressions, good or bad, may set the course for future sexual encounters.

Although sex would seem inherently pleasurable, religious and cultural prohibitions can conspire to restrict its enjoyment through guilt or punishment. Negative associations, fostered in childhood, can create conflicting feelings that interfere with successful sexual functioning in the adult. Adults who were sexually abused as children are an extreme example of this kind of problem. Likewise, a string of sexual experiences in which a man has received negative feedback—from a partner frustrated with his poor erectile performance, for example—can make sex unattractive, leading to low desire or worsening problems with erections.

If your experience with sex has been positive, then you look forward to future sexual encounters with a sense of pleasurable anticipation. Dissatisfying or unpleasant sex, or an upbringing that characterized sex as dirty or shameful, can create a psychological pattern that interferes with healthy sexual functioning. Sex therapists can help you and your partner overcome a history of less-than-satisfying sexual experiences.

Unfortunately, a history of positive feelings surrounding one's sexual education and experiences isn't an ironclad guarantee that problems won't arise in the future. As you'll see in the case of Jim and Mary Campbell, later in this chapter, a completely problem-free history creates its own difficulties—when a crisis does arise, the participants may be devastated. Since nothing in their history has prepared them for trouble, it comes as that much greater a shock. But, here too, as you'll see, the guidance of a therapist can turn devastation into a renewed commitment for the couple involved.

STRESS, ANXIETY AND FATIGUE

Good erectile physiology, the right sensory stimulation and a history of positive sexual experiences can still be undermined by abnormal psychological factors. Sex researchers have identified a group of emotional variables that, taken together, tend to inhibit sexual feelings.

Most of these variables are connected with stress, along with the more common emotional responses to stress—anxiety and fatigue. Depression can also be a stress response and can also complicate matters.

That stress negatively affects our thoughts, feelings and physical condition is well established. Exactly how stress will affect *your* erections depends on your psychological and physical makeup.

Stress may lead to increased circulating blood levels of *adrenaline* and activation of nerves to the penis that release the neurotransmitter *noradrenaline* (the sympathetic nerves). Both of these effects adversely influence erections by causing smooth-muscle tissue to constrict in the penis's arteries and by preventing the relaxation of the smooth muscle surrounding the lacunar spaces in the penis (see illustration, page 13).

In addition, when we become preoccupied with work or family or money, to cite the most common sources of stress, worrisome thoughts override sexual stimulation; we don't become aroused as easily. As family or money troubles demand more and more of our attention, we may spend more and more time trying to think of solutions for our problems. Preoccupation with these difficulties may crowd out "less important" concerns in a couple's life, like sexual desire. Just about every popular news magazine these days has devoted space to the too-tired-to-make-love syndrome among upwardly mobile couples whose hard-driving lifestyles have shoved aside room for true intimacy. It's hardly surprising that sex under such pressured circumstances isn't rewarding; intimacy can't be turned on or off at a moment's notice — it needs cultivation. It's not unusual for such couples to end up avoiding sex as a means of eliminating one more pressured area in their lives. But such avoidance can, over time, destroy a relationship.

———— ♦ ————

Anxiety can either be remote from sex itself or connected to the sexual situation. If you're preoccupied with trouble at your workplace or worried about caring for an ill parent, you may have trouble becoming aroused.

In the same way, anxiety that centers around sexual performance itself, sometimes called *performance anxiety*, can interfere with enjoyment. The message from films and television is that all men are — or should be — capable of becoming aroused on cue, so it's not surprising that performance anxiety is a routine complaint in sex therapists' offices.

Fears about AIDS and other diseases, fear of pregnancy and fear of intimacy commonly inhibit arousal, as do resentment toward one's partner or toward women or men in general. Feelings of shame or guilt, either left over from one's upbringing, or related to a specific sexual situation (an instance of infidelity, for example) are other frequently cited sources of inhibition of sexual responsiveness.

Anxiety is a common but powerful deterrent to a good sexual relationship. Fortunately, sex therapists have made great strides in treating anxiety-based sexual dysfunction.

DEPRESSION

Depression, like anxiety, may be either the result or the cause of impotence. People suffering from depression typically lose interest in those things in life that give pleasure. Lack of interest in sex, in fact, is often regarded as a major symptom of depression. By the same token, men who are impotent tend to get depressed about it, and so set themselves up on a vicious cycle.

Studies have shown that depressed people regard life pessimistically; they anticipate the worst in any outcome, and they focus more on negative experiences than on positive ones. Consequently, a man suffering from a depression due to nonsexual events can easily find himself triggering his own impotence. First, he anticipates his own poor performance, then fulfills his own prophecy by making himself too anxious to become aroused; subsequent negative anticipations lead to further failure, and ultimately to avoidance of sex altogether.

A type of treatment called *cognitive behavioral therapy* has been designed to specifically combat the continual negative reinforcement to which mildly depressed or anxious patients subject themselves. In this type of therapy, patients are taught to identify and challenge negative thinking. For example, in place of "I know my erection won't last," a man might substitute, "Even if we don't have intercourse it will still feel good to cuddle and caress." By learning to challenge negative thoughts and avoid dwelling on their fears, patients gain control of their emotional state.

Sex Therapy

As recently as twenty years ago, a man suffering from impotence had few places where he could find help to determine whether his problem was physical or psychological. The common medical view was that if a man wasn't getting proper erections, he either needed more testosterone or help with the emotional disturbance that must be the root of his problem. Twenty years ago a common answer was psychoanalysis.

Psychoanalysis was time-consuming, expensive and, given the recent insights into erectile physiology, often ineffective. The goal was to bring to light the repressed contents of the impotent man's unconscious mind; as these hidden conflicts emerged into awareness and were faced by the patient, so the theory held, the sexual symptoms associated with their repression, including impotence, would disappear. In the closed world of psychoanalytic theory, however, the search for the ultimate hidden conflict, the one that would liberate the patient's captive potency, often became a neverending quest for the psychic Holy Grail.

Psychoanalysis made no provision for a man with a damaged circulatory system in his penis. If a man's penis refused to become erect, it was interpreted as a sure sign of his "resistance" to therapy, and more therapy was needed. Analysis, whatever its other merits, was clearly not suitable as a treatment for the overwhelming majority of impotent men, but for many years it was almost the only option available.

Pioneers of sex research like Drs. William Masters and Virginia Johnson, soon followed by Dr. Helen Singer Kaplan, revolutionized the treatment of impotence in the 1970s by developing short-term, highly focused approaches to problems of sexual function. Instead of rooting about in the patients' unconscious minds, the exercises directly addressed the feelings and behavior of the couple in a sexual situation.

Masters' and Johnson's most well-known contribution to the field of sex therapy is a series of exercises called *sensate focus*, which I mentioned earlier. The exercises engage both members of a couple in the therapeutic process. Practicing at home, each partner takes turns giving and receiving pleasure. The receiver communicates in a noncritical way what he or she prefers. The giver obliges as much as possible. The couple then visits their sex therapist to report on their "homework."

Different exercises are used to address different problems–premature ejaculation, say, requires the couple to adjust their behavior in ways different from the treatment for erectile insufficiency–but the graduated nature of the exercises is common to all of them. In treating a case of pyschogenic impotence, for example, a couple might spend several weeks on nonsexual touching and massage, later introducing erotic elements into their encounters in small, nonthreatening steps, only moving to intercourse toward the very end of their treatment.

At present, sensate focus exercises are just one of an expanded set of techniques now available to therapists and their clients. These include a repertoire of short-term approaches, as well as the more traditional "talking therapies," used to address relationship problems or deeply rooted personality disorders.

HOW THERAPY WORKS

The traditional Masters-and-Johnson approach to sex therapy utilized couples, composed of one male and one female therapist, but today therapists may just as likely operate alone as with one or more other health professionals. They may also be part of a larger group practice, as in a university-affiliated impotence clinic, where the group might also include a urologist and an endocrinologist.

In addressing the psychological side of impotence, therapists by and large prefer to see both members of a couple, rather than just the man. Most psychogenic impotence is situational. That is, it arises out of feelings and behavior connected with a specific sexual relationship. When a man has trouble with his erections, the problem is a shared one; the relationship—not just the man and his erections —suffers. The sexual interaction in a relationship, a complicated dance in the best of times, is often a major part of the problem. Unknowingly, each dancer may be communicating the wrong signals to his or her partner. By dealing with impotence as a couple, the partners can sort through these signals in an environment that makes the goal of therapy the restoration of the couple's sexual well-being, rather than assigning blame or "taking care of his problem."

Given the astonishing breadth of variation among all the factors that affect our sexual functioning—age, upbringing, religious and cultural factors—it shouldn't be surprising that different couples require different kinds of therapy for different lengths of time.

Occasionally, all that is necessary to restore a couple to happy functioning is for a figure of professional authority, the sex therapist, to give the clients "permission" to enjoy their sexuality or offer assurance that "they're normal."

I'll give you a couple of examples from my own practice. (The biographical details of cases have been changed to protect privacy.)

———— ◆ ————

During intercourse with his girlfriend, a patient of mine suddenly imagined her humiliating him. The fantasy shocked him and left him disturbed for several days afterward. He wondered if he was "perverted," or if the simple act of envisioning such a scene would compel him to act it out in real life. The next time he tried to make love, his guilt and concern interfered with his ability to relax, and he couldn't get an erection.

Much has been written about unusual or bizarre fantasies during sex. Husbands and wives who wouldn't dream of breaking their marriage vows take imaginary lovers themselves or imagine their mates with them. Violence or pain may figure in the picture. The unexpected appearance of one of these mental scenarios can feel quite threatening, especially if it doesn't conform to our ideas of how we ought to behave. We fear fantasies precisely because they often include activities that are illegal or would invite social disapproval.

But unless the fantasy becomes obsessional or the exclusive focus of one's erotic fulfillment, it needn't disrupt intimacy.

I informed the man that simply having the humiliation fantasy did not mean that he had to act on it, any more than any of us has to act on any of the other fantasies which pervade our lives. With this information, the patient no longer felt he was losing control of his life. Now, when he has fantasies like this, he notices them—and lets them go—without letting them disrupt his lovemaking.

Another of my patients, a shy young man with little sexual experience, attended a large university, where he met a young woman and fell in love. His previous sexual encounters had been with high-school girlfriends who passively "let him fool around," with no evident enjoyment on their part. His college girlfriend, more experienced than he, suggested they spend a night together. With a mixture of guilt and eagerness, he agreed.

Her lack of inhibition once they were in bed intimidated him, and, too embarrassed to admit he was still a virgin, he lost his erection.

I was able to reassure this young man that an enthusiastic expression of sexuality, by men and women, is a normal part of a healthy relationship. That was all the reassurance he needed.

———— ♦ ————

The majority of couples require more intervention than the above examples, often using one of the programs of structured exercises. Multiple episodes of impotence usually indicate that the couple stands to benefit by setting a series of goals designed to enhance their relationship. These goals include:

Establishing mutual responsibility for satisfaction. From the perspective of the therapist, the relationship between the two partners is the problem. Impotence—or for that matter, any problem with sexual functioning—is a shared problem. Individual blame is minimized, and a spirit of cooperation is fostered.

Correcting myths and misinformation. This information may involve informing the couples about sexual physiology or correcting myths about sexuality, for example. Once in a while, as in the cases discussed above, providing information will, by itself, take care of the problem. More often, correcting misinformation is an adjunct to other kinds of therapeutic approaches.

Ensuring that the couples receive a high level of physical and psychological stimulation. Generally, this is accomplished by expanding the couple's sexual repertoire and improving their communication in sexual matters. Sometimes, poor communications skills between partners lead to mistaken beliefs about each other's attitudes and reactions. Sensate focus exercises, in teaching couples how to give and receive pleasure, and how to communicate sexually, encourage couples to explore their sexuality in a gradual, non-threatening manner. Partners learn how to ask for what excites them most, how to accommodate each other's changing moods and address each other's sexual needs. The therapist can also help partners to express themselves verbally, and can recommend books that provide techniques for improving communication.

Eliminating mental distractions. Mental static in the form of "spectatoring" (watching your own lovemaking to see how you're doing), negative thoughts and anxiety about sexual performance can chill the arousal of the most hot-blooded lover. Even positive distracting thoughts can interfere with sex. A man who can't keep his mind off an anticipated promotion may have as much trouble functioning as another man who's obsessed with losing his job. The point is, you can't watch two channels at once and expect to have satisfying sex. Structured exercises can help clients relax and stay positively focused on lovemaking. Treatment may also include learning muscle relaxation and a technique called *systematic desensitization*, the pairing of relaxation with sexual images or situations. Also, by taking turns in the sensate focus exercises, the impotent man can learn to relax and enjoy himself without worrying about his partner's satisfaction.

Eliminating relationship interference. Marital tension seldom stops at the bedroom door. If a couple can't communicate their general needs and desires, if they can't resolve the conflicts which inevitably arise in daily life, there's little reason to think that they're going to be able to accomplish with sex what they fail to do in other (often less threatening) areas of behavior. In such cases the sex therapist may suggest training in family dynamics and in communications and conflict-resolution skills, as a useful addition to the sexually focused work.

IS SEX THERAPY FOR YOU?

Discussing your sex life with a stranger, even a professionally sanctioned stranger, can be an unnerving task. The people who gain most from this type of therapy usually do so because of their willingness to articulate their feelings and to set aside previous patterns of behavior and prejudices. Therapists understand the delicacy of their task and will help you over the initial inhibitions of discussion, but you must cooperate as well. Communication between all the people in the process—you, your partner and the therapist(s)—is crucial. If you're open to the idea of such discussion, despite some initial reservations, you may benefit from therapy.

An accommodating partner is critical. Most therapy is designed for couples, since most sexual problems occur within the context of a relationship. A supportive partner facilitates the changes in attitudes or technique necessary to restoring successful sexual intimacy.

An uncaring partner, or one unwilling to address his or her own role in the sexual relationship, makes the goals of sex therapy more difficult to achieve.

Sometimes, unsure what to expect, a man will come alone to his initial session of therapy, with instructions from his spouse or girlfriend to "check out the situation." Once the woman is assured of the professional approach and environment, she will often agree to join in the process.

Some therapists suggest that you postpone sex therapy if you're having marital problems that extend beyond the sexual sphere. Otherwise, relationship issues may mask themselves as sexual difficulties. I suggest that people engage in both types of therapy (marital and sexual) at once. The sex therapist should also be skilled in couple therapy or family therapy. If you haven't a solid base of intimacy on which the relationship rests, it's unlikely that sex therapy alone will magically give it to you. But if you're committed to establishing intimacy, and working hard at doing so, sex therapy can be a valuable adjunct in extending that process into what is for many couples the most sensitive part of their relationship.

Some of you may be wondering, can you have sex therapy if you don't have a partner? At one time, Masters and Johnson utilized sexual surrogates, women who were paid to act as partners for single men. Many other clinics followed suit. The use of surrogates has always been controversial, with opposed therapists claiming that their use is neither effective nor moral. To the best of our knowledge, the use of surrogates has been condemned by the American Pyschological Association.

My own feeling is that a single man with psychogenic impotence is best served by working with a therapist to develop his social skills before concentrating on his sexual problems. Once he's established a relationship with a partner, he can invite her to participate in sex therapy with him. Some therapists are willing to prescribe exercises for the single man that combine masturbation with visualization, but these obviously have their limitations.

There are some other factors to consider when making a decision about sex therapy. Substance abuse, increasingly common in our society, may affect your decision—or the therapist's. Heavy intake of alcohol or drugs like cocaine interferes with sexual functioning, blurring the physiological effects of the abuse with the patient's own psychology. Most therapists will decline to treat alcoholics or drug abusers with sex therapy until the issue of substance abuse has been addressed and a period of detoxification of six months has elapsed.

Certain types of mental illness, like severe depression or anxiety disorders, may also make people unsuitable for sex therapy, because patient and therapist have difficulty distinguishing feelings connected with sexual functioning from those related to the primary illness. Mild anxiety and depression, however, can often improve after sex therapy, and should not pose a barrier to seeking therapy.

CHOOSING A SEX THERAPIST— WHAT TO LOOK FOR

A urologist specializing in impotence should be able to recommend sex therapists in your area. Family physicians, local hospitals, even the yellow pages of your phone book, list therapists who treat sexual problems. Large urban areas often offer psychotherapy referral services that can also direct you.

It's a good idea to start with the names of several therapists—in the event that for any reason you're not comfortable with one, you can interview one or two more before committing yourself to treatment.

Qualified sex therapists come in all shades of academic accreditation. The American Association of Sex Educators, Counselors and Therapists (AASECT) certifies professionals who meet its standards of training and education, but not all therapists are officially certified. The American Board of Family Psychology also requires its members to meet specific criteria before certifying them as sex therapists, but again, not all psychologists who practice sex therapy are certified by these organizations. Other sources of credentials may be memberships on the staff of a hospital, teaching facility, clinic or health maintenance organization (HMO).

As a consumer, you should be aware that the term "sex therapist" carries no guarantees of any sort—except that the person who claims the title is willing to treat you. He or she may be a medical doctor, a psychologist, a social worker or a nurse—or have no training in health care or counseling at all. For this reason, you need to exercise more than usual vigilance when choosing a therapist, especially one who comes without a personal recommendation. All qualified therapists will willingly answer your questions. If the therapist is evasive or refuses to answer your questions, leave.

You should ask your therapist about his or her educational background and, specifically, where he got his or her training in sex therapy. The therapist should be licensed in his or her field, such as psychology, nursing or social work, if not in sex therapy itself. Each state has licensing boards that oversee each of the various disciplines. For example, if your therapist is a social worker, he or she should be licensed in your state; the same holds true for psychologists, psychiatrists and nurses. (A few states use the term "certification" instead of the term "licensure." Usually, boards of health care professionals "certify" and state authorities "license." State requirements, whatever they're called, are usually stricter than those of professional boards.)

During your first interview you can learn much about your therapist just by noting what sort of questions you're asked. At the very least, your therapist should question you about your general health and the medical tests and treatments you've undergone so far. He or she should ask for the name of your urologist and ask to see the results of your examination. At the very least, he or she should demonstrate a familiarity with the tests and procedures used by your urologist.

You should be asked specific, explicit questions concerning your sexual functioning. Good therapists try to establish the exact circumstances surrounding a particular problem. To do this they need to establish an accurate portrait of your behavior before, during and after the problem occurred. Your partner should also be interviewed. Some therapists prefer to speak with partners separately during the first visit; others like to interview them together because it gives the therapist an immediate overall glimpse of the partners' relationship.

Since treatment of sexual problems can involve a wide range of options, from short-term, highly focused exercises to intensive psychotherapy, ask the therapist for the range of his or her own treatment methods. Some therapists prefer to specialize in cases amenable to short-term treatment; others center the bulk of their practice on long-term marital psychotherapy. The best therapists can do both, as needed by their clients.

Also, ask whether he or she has ever dealt with your problem before. If so, how frequently?

No ethical therapist will ever propose a treatment that involves sex between the therapist and you—or the therapist and anyone else. If a therapist proposes or initiates sex, leave at once and report the therapist to the state licensing board that covers your therapist. Such behavior is considered a violation of the professional code of ethics of the American Psychological Association. Sex between therapist and clients is almost always exploitive of the patient, with no therapeutic value.

In some cases a single interview with both members of a couple present may be all that's required for a therapist to form a diagnosis and propose a treatment plan. For impotence, however, it's more than likely that the initial interviews will require at least two visits. The therapist will want a thorough knowledge of the client's medical background and any treatment or medication he might be taking that could affect his potency. He or she will also want an extensive grounding in the couple's sexual history.

By the third visit, the therapist should offer you a diagnosis and a treatment plan. He or she should explain his or her own role in the treatment and outline how you and your partner will be expected to participate. The therapist should also estimate how long the treatment will last and how much it will cost.

Since some clinics offer standardized programs of treatment for specific problems (e.g., a thirty-visit series, lasting four months, for erectile problems) you should find out the payment policy if for some reason you need to stop treatment. You should also check the extent of your insurance coverage for sex therapy.

Assuming the therapist seems qualified, the final question to ask is whether you and your partner feel comfortable with him or her. Even short-term therapy gives rise to strong feelings that, if not shared with your therapist, can undermine your treatment. It's critical that you settle on a therapist with whom you can build a trusting relationship.

Jim and Mary— A Case of Psychogenic Impotence

The following is a close look at one couple's experience with sex therapy. Jim and Mary Campbell (not their real names) were a middle-class couple in their early forties when they came to my office. For the five months prior to seeking therapy, Jim had been experiencing frequent problems with his erections. He had visited a urologist, who found no evidence of organic damage to his erectile system. During their first visit, I interviewed them together, obtaining their pertinent sex histories and the evolution of their problem. Their therapy lasted for sixteen sessions over about four months and was highly successful.

A HAPPY MARRIAGE

The Campbells had been married eighteen years and had three children, all in high school. Both of them worked. Jim was a midlevel manager for a pharmaceuticals firm. Mary, who had earned a master's degree while raising their children, had resumed her career as a special education instructor. Except for this recent disruption in their sex life, they described themselves as highly compatible and their marriage as having been a happy one.

Both Jim and Mary came from religious families whose values disapproved of premarital sex. They met in high school, were attracted and became chaste sweethearts. After graduation, they separated for a few years, attending different colleges. Both of them dated in college, but neither was yet sexually active. A chance meeting during vacation between their junior and senior years rekindled their romance and they became engaged the following Christmas.

Both of them came to the marriage as virgins, acquiring their sexual know-how through a reasonably successful process of trial and error.

Jim had a tendency in the early stage of their marriage to ejaculate prematurely, leaving Mary frustrated and unsatisfied. But he trained himself to postpone his ejaculation until Mary had received sufficient stimulation to reach her own orgasm. They described their sexual relationship over the course of their marriage as intensely gratifying. For several years previous to visiting me, they had sex two or three times a week, a pattern that satisfied both of them.

AN ANXIOUS WATCHFULNESS

Several months ago they had gone to the Caribbean for a week-long vacation without their children. They sailed, relaxed on the beach and in the late afternoons made love with wild abandon. But towards the end of the week, Jim became preoccupied with a work problem he'd left unresolved before leaving on vacation. On the last day of their trip, they went back to their bungalow for a final afternoon of lovemaking. This time, however, Jim failed to become erect.

This had never happened before.

Neither of them became upset. It was, they told themselves, "just one of those things." They readily admitted that Jim was under a fair amount of stress. His recent career change had taken him from a small company to a large one. His new job was much more demanding job than his previous one, involving a promotion and greater responsibility. He had been at his previous job for seven years, had liked the people and felt safe and comfortable. The new job paid much more, but his head, as he expressed it, was never far from the chopping block.

When they came back from vacation they fell into their normal routine of sex two or three times a week. But, a month later, Jim again failed to become erect.

This time they were seized with panic. Jim was mortified and Mary felt incompetent. An anxious watchfulness soon pervaded their lovemaking—and Jim failed to become erect the next three times in a row. Their lovemaking, and his erections, had been sporadic ever since.

Jim's impotence plunged their relationship into an emotional tailspin. Mary gained weight; Jim became preoccupied with his work. For the first time in their married lives, they began to seriously ask themselves whether they had misjudged themselves. Maybe they really weren't intended for each other—a fear that terrified both of them.

SENSATE FOCUS EXERCISES

Even without the exact specifics of their interactions, which I would learn in the following weeks, it wasn't difficult to see how Jim and Mary had psychologically painted themselves into a corner. The success or failure of their marriage had come to depend on whether they successfully managed to have intercourse. No wonder Jim was so infrequently aroused—he was worried about the consequences of what would happen if he didn't become excited.

I defused some of their anxiety by telling them that all marriages go through crises—every seven to ten years, according to some studies. Nor does a crisis necessarily spell the end of a relationship. In fact, it can often lead to a renewed sense of commitment in a couple.

I explained how a program of sensate focus exercises would help identify problematic areas in their sexual relationship, which we could discuss during office visits. At the same time, the exercises would begin restoring the intimacy which had been so damaged by their recent problem.

They agreed to give the program a try.

Jim and Mary's first homework assignment was to engage in nongenital caressing—back rubs, neck rubs, body massage. They would report back to me in a week. I emphasized that the goal of the assignment was *not* to give Jim an erection. If his penis became erect, fine. If he didn't have an erection, that was also fine. In the meantime, I asked them to refrain from any overt sexual contact, especially intercourse. Each time they had tried to have intercourse— and failed—it had contributed to their history of negative sexual experiences.

Sensate focus exercises offer couples an avenue out of the charged arena of dysfunctional sex. The program asks them to put their present difficulties on hold, and return to basics, the simple giving and receiving of pleasure.

In the beginning, that pleasure is *nonsexual*. A clear understanding is reached that no attempts will be made to have intercourse or to achieve orgasm. The couple is encouraged to provide sensuous pleasure for each other, alternating the giving and receiving roles.

In the first exercises, breast and genital touching is prohibited. If arousal occurs, it is to be ignored. In subsequent pleasuring sessions, stroking of the genitals is permitted with continued restrictions on intercourse or orgasm. The goal of this therapy is to enable the couple to learn that erections will occur during relaxed play, that if the erection subsides another may occur and that intercourse is not necessary each time arousal occurs. The message is: You don't have to do anything sexual, so how can you fail?

As the weeks pass, and the couple becomes accustomed to making love without having to meet anyone's performance standards, the partners' own erotic instincts begin to emerge. As the couple grows more confident, the man is instructed to insert his penis into the woman with the woman on top. First, this is done without movement. Then, gradually increasing stimulation is added with slow and then more vigorous thrusting.

Couples are usually instructed to stop stimulating each other before either of them reaches orgasm. Each session ends with desire still smoldering. Sex therapy can be said to have succeeded when a couple's own hunger for their next sexual encounter displaces their previous anxious anticipation of it.

Like many couples, Jim and Mary had assumed that each of them was supposed to know intuitively exactly what the other wanted, and even exactly how the other person felt. But by trying to be Mr. and Ms. Perfect, and expecting the same from the other, they were bound to be disappointed.

No one knows better than you what you want or feel. If you want something, you can help your partner be more perfect, more wonderful, by simply saying what you want and assuming responsibility for your own satisfaction. By telling the other person, you are sharing responsibility.

The exercises were designed in part to teach Jim and Mary how to ask each other for what they wanted.

The exercises were also designed to teach Jim and Mary that arousal comes and goes. Just because Jim loses his arousal one minute doesn't mean that it won't be back the next minute.

They would also learn how to be "in the moment" during their sensual encounters — to agree, at least for the time of their lovemaking, to concentrate on just enjoying one another without interference from the stresses of life which otherwise occupied them.

Finally, doing the exercises would help them reinforce their commitment to the relationship. Instead of "Uh-oh, Jim can't get an erection," the exercises helped them reframe the problem, to think, "The intimate side of our relationship has run into a snag—both of us are working on untangling it."

At our second meeting, a week later, Jim and Mary reported on their progress. They had each taken turns giving and receiving massage, as instructed. The first session had been a success. Mary's reminders to Jim that all he had to do was enjoy himself had helped him overcome his initial anxiety. No one was requiring him to get an erection. As soon as he relaxed, his penis became erect. They confided that this had so excited both of them that they had briefly ignored the prohibition against genital caressing.

The next session, however, had been a disappointment. After their first success, Jim expected he would become excited right away. When he didn't, he became discouraged and anxious.

Part of my instruction during their first visit had been that they share their anxieties with each other as they occurred. During their second visit, however, it became clear to me that both of them were too wrapped up in their respective anxieties to yet be of much help to each other. I spent twenty minutes with each of them alone, eliciting descriptions of their separate fears.

Jim confessed that during much of the sensate focus sessions his thoughts would become a veritable babble of dire predictions: I'm never going to be able to make love to Mary again; I'm always disappointing her; she's going to leave me for another man; our marriage is over, etc.

For her part, Mary was uncomfortable with Jim's sudden dependence on her. She was the sort of person who rarely said no. The world made many demands on her, which she readily accepted, knowing that she could count on Jim for emotional support. She volunteered time out of her busy schedule for church activities.

When one of their children needed a parent to participate in a school activity, Mary was the one to go. Jim worked long hours that often prevented him from filling these roles. Throughout their marriage, that had been fine with Mary. Jim, independent and calm, was always willing to lend an ear when she became too frustrated — and Mary had leaned on him. When Jim suddenly stepped out of his traditional role by asking her to reassure him that he was OK as a man, the balance in their relationship shifted. She felt betrayed and angry. If Jim, her rock and support, began clinging to her, where was she to go for her own psychic nourishment? The more dependent he became, the more she freaked out. She began pushing him away, confirming his worst fears.

As Jim and Mary talked, it became evident that this was a time of intense transition for them. Their children were growing up, Mary's schedule was changing with her return to teaching, and Jim was under intense pressure to prove himself at work. Now on top of all this, their love life had become shaky.

Transitions — personal and professional — are a time of tremendous psychological upheaval. Anxieties established early in our family backgrounds, normally not evident, come to the fore, making us vulnerable in previously unsuspected ways.

When Jim failed to have an erection, it triggered a crisis in Mary's mind. She began overeating. Mary's father had been very critical of her mother's appearance. Whenever her mother had put on weight,

Mary's father had threatened to leave her. Mary now feared that Jim no longer found her attractive, and that he would take the same attitude as her father.

Jim had his own demons from the past that needed examination. His parents had not been not been physically or emotionally close. They had never hugged or kissed in public, and Jim had no doubt that this coolness extended to the bedroom as well. By contrast, the physical dimension of his own marriage was something he relished. Now he started anticipating a replication of his parents' loveless marriage.

OVERCOMING ANXIETY
AND MISCOMMUNICATION

The psychological forces in Jim and Mary's relationship revealed themselves through their descriptions of their thoughts during anxious moments in their sensate focus sessions. After listening to them individually and together, I concluded that neither of them was ready to offer each other much emotional support. They were too anxious.

Their first tasks, then, were to learn how to calm down, how to substitute reality for their understandable, but unrealistic, fears and how to express their needs to each other.

First, I instructed them in techniques for progressive muscle relaxation. I included these instructions on a tape, which Jim, as the most anxious of the two, would use twice a day. Listening to the tape, Jim would practice relaxing, beginning with his toes, alternately tensing and relaxing them, moving through all the muscle groups in his body, matching his breathing to his muscle movements. Instead of trying to push anxious thoughts away, he was instructed to redirect his attention back to his breath and his body whenever a threatening image came up.

Ultimately, as this technique for redirecting his attention became automatic, Jim would be able to use it when he became anxious during sensate focus with Mary.

I also instructed Jim to prepare a set of affirmative phrases he could use to combat anxious thoughts. When, for example, the thought that Mary was going to leave him arose, he would repeat to himself, "I can't predict the future. Mary's here because she loves me. I'm just going to enjoy being with her now." Substituting affirmative thoughts in place of negative ones is a form of reality checking. Jim's wife wasn't about to leave him — and he needed to tell himself so.

Mary's anxiety lessened just by seeing Jim begin to take responsibility for managing his fears himself, instead of relying on her alone. I explained to her that "dry spells" in marriages are not unusual, and that in her own case it certainly didn't seem to signal a decline in her appeal for Jim. Dry spells often arrive in times of stress, and depart soon after. She was encouraged to engage in her own reality checking and to develop her own reality affirmations. Jim loved her. She was attractive and sexy. They were working it out.

In the beginning of their treatment, they often surprised each other as they began to express themselves honestly. Mary was amazed to learn that Jim wasn't in the least concerned that she'd put on a little extra weight.

For his part, Jim was surprised to hear that Mary would willingly consider introducing mutual masturbation and oral sex into their sexual repertoire, not just as precursors to intercourse, but as satisfying alternatives to it. "I didn't think you'd like that!" he protested. "You just never asked," she replied.

Jim and Mary's relationship impressed me as basically sound. Their ability to share an important aspect of their lives had temporarily gotten off track, undoubtedly a frightening experience for both of them, but not one which would sink their marriage. I was convinced that if they could manage to gain some control over their fears, then the positive aspects of their relationship would reassert themselves.

To this end, for the next couple of weeks they were directed to concentrate on reducing their anxiety through the exercises described above.

I also departed from a strict adherence to the structures of sensate focus and concentrated instead on restoring some of their day-to-day intimacies.

In the charged atmosphere of their crisis, for example, Mary had come to dread, and then to avoid altogether, Jim's morning good-bye kiss. Before leaving for work he would cling to her like a soldier leaving for the front; at night, the procedure reversed itself, and he would hug her like a man miraculously afforded one last reprieve against the inevitable departure of his wife. Now they were encouraged to resume their hugging and kissing, and if they became uncomfortable, to remember their reality affirmations.

The major areas of miscommunication between Jim and Mary became clear after four or five visits. Their anxieties visibly diminished within two weeks of beginning to practice reality checking and muscle relaxation, and they eagerly resumed sensate focus, moving from nonsexual massage to genital caressing.

Both of them were learning how to express themselves in a new language. Before Jim's impotence, their lovemaking had always followed the same pattern of foreplay culminating in intercourse. Now they were encouraged to give and receive sexual pleasure without intercourse.

While playing the role of receiver, each of them had to learn to explicitly communicate his or her needs, to receive pleasure without worrying about the other person; in the role of giver, they each had to learn to respond to their partner as fully as possible, without worrying about themselves.

Jim and Mary learned to communicate what relaxed and what aroused each of them. People often have an idealized image of sex, of being carried away by the excitement of the moment, both partners wordlessly stimulating and encouraging each other until they explode in mutual orgasm. Stars flash and bells ring. Sometimes this happens — but lots of times it doesn't. A great sexual relationship is more often the result of flexibility, patience and forthright communication than coincidence.

This couple had been coasting for years — they'd found something that worked for them and they'd stuck with it. Many couples operate this way. The inherent weakness of such an arrangement is that if something disrupts the couple's life, they then lack the tools to address the problem and repair it.

Sex therapy wasn't "solving" Jim and Mary's problem — it was teaching them a process, a way of communicating with each other that would enable them to solve it themselves. They were taking responsibility for their own sexual satisfaction.

TRUSTING INSIGHTS

Jim and Mary's therapy lasted a total of sixteen sessions over about four months. Their deepest insights about their own behavior came quite early in the process, which is not unusual. Most of the therapy was devoted to teaching them to *trust* those insights — that their marriage wasn't coming to an end, that they loved each other, that they could communicate their sexual likes and dislikes openly, without shame or fear, and that they could successfully take responsibility for how they felt.

A distinct change came over their demeanor as their anxiety lessened. Instead of listening apprehensively to each other's comments on how the sessions had gone, they listened neutrally, then with humor.

Jim and Mary did have setbacks during the course of treatment. Fortunately, they realized that setbacks can be an important tool for achieving success in the long run. By overcoming setbacks, you gain confidence in your own abilities to become aroused.

One of Jim's setbacks occurred after he had started getting regular erections. His erections resumed with such regularity that he assumed he'd never have a problem again. Of course, an occasion did come up when penis failed to get erect as quickly as it had previously. He was immediately filled with despair. He believed everything he'd worked so hard to attain during the first ten weeks of therapy was obviously gone. All the old thoughts about Mary leaving him boiled up in his head again, and for a second he felt overwhelmed.

At our next session I had to remind him to return to repeating his reality affirmations. Erections come and go; his erections would be back again. He was soon able to get back to lovemaking. What would have been a crisis several months before was only a momentary interruption now.

I knew Jim and Mary's therapy was almost at an end when they began groping for things to talk about during our visits. They often smiled at my questions, like people sharing an inside joke, and they held hands. The day arrived when they giggled and confessed that they'd broken my rule and gone ahead and had intercourse. Twice. They were sorry, but they just couldn't help themselves. Many therapists never tell their clients to have intercourse—I certainly didn't with Jim and Mary.

They'd done the right thing, I assured them. Lovers themselves, not therapists, should decide when they're ready to make the leap.

I met with Jim and Mary once more, then scheduled a follow-up visit four months later. They were calm and happy. Jim seemed to have settled into his job, and the worry that had weighed them down in our first meeting had completely vanished. They were doing fine, Mary said, and Jim nodded agreement.

"You didn't cure us—we did," Mary said. "But we couldn't have done it without learning some new tools for our marriage. If it happens again, we'll be prepared, not threatened."

Success Stories

———— ◆ ————

In the next four chapters, you'll read about four men with organic impotence who were treated at our impotence clinic at Boston University Medical Center. Three of these patients underwent surgery and one uses injection therapy. At our institution, we treat impotence as conservatively as possible, using such treatments as sex therapy, vacuum constriction device therapy or injection therapy initially and performing surgery only when necessary. Patients who need surgery are encouraged to discuss their fears and concerns with me, my staff and, if necessary, with sex therapist Alma Dell Smith.

Each of the stories in chapters 4 through 7 includes the patient's own narrative about his diagnosis and treatment, my comments about the patient's diagnosis and treatment and the comments of Dr. Alma Dell Smith concerning the psychological aspects of each case. Dr. Smith's analyses are based on the patients' histories and taped interviews as well as, in some cases, her own evaluation of or therapy with the patients.

–Irwin Goldstein, M.D.

———— ◆ ————

CHAPTER 4

Tom — A Surgical Success Story

When Tom Killian (not his real name) came to our clinic, he was thirty-nine years old, recently remarried and employed as a hospital lab technician. That was in the early spring of 1984. His erectile insufficiency was caused by a "failure to fill." His potency was restored in a surgical procedure known as revascularization, *which means the rerouting of blood vessels. It is also called* arterial bypass *surgery. An artery from Tom's abdominal wall was rerouted and connected to two arteries in his penis. In this chapter, and the following one, I discuss the rapid surgical advances that have been made in the last several years in surgery for impotence.*

Tom's Story

From the time I first made love at fourteen until I was thirty-seven, I never had any sexual problems beyond occasional impotence due to drinking or fatigue. For most of my life I've been known as a ladies' man. It was a large part of my identity. I didn't go around bragging, but other people knew of it and blew it out of proportion. Friends would sometimes introduce me as "Tom the Lover."

I was married at twenty-eight and divorced at thirty-three. I have a six-year-old son named Tom, Jr., whom I see on weekends.

I'd been dating for five years without becoming seriously involved with anyone until I met Nancy. She was thirty-two when we met, divorced and living with her five-year-old daughter, Carrie. She worked as an executive secretary for a stock brokerage firm.

It was strange. Right after I met Nancy I began to have these impotence problems. Here I was, this virile man always capable of doing whatever I wanted to do sexually, and then all of a sudden I couldn't. Sometimes someone would look at me and I'd think, I wonder if they know . . . I wonder if I have that look that I can't get it up. Is there a look? Is there something I'm doing, some sort of vibration that I'm giving off so that they know that I'm impotent? I wondered that many, many times. I never knew the answer.

COULDN'T PERFORM

I first met Nancy in the spring of 1983 at a sports bar in downtown Boston. We started talking while we watched the Red Sox play on the bar's television. We hit it off almost from the beginning. I had more fun with her than with any girl that I had met in a long time. After a couple of dates, we went home to her apartment and I tried to make love to Nancy but I just couldn't perform. Nancy asked me what was wrong and I said, "I'm not sure. But I'll be all right. This happens once in a while." I shrugged it off as opening-night jitters. Nancy was more upset, however. She started to cry. She told me this was her first sexual experience since her divorce, and that she had never known anyone else but her husband. Nancy thought she was doing something wrong, that she wasn't turning me on. I assured her that it wasn't her fault. We held each other closely that night until we fell asleep.

A week later the same thing happened. This time I got a little anxious. I didn't understand this. I was certainly attracted to her. I started to rationalize that maybe it had to do with her still living in the same house where she had been married. I told Nancy maybe there's a sense of past history that's working on me that I'm not really conscious of. I suggested that we go away for the weekend and take the pressure off both of us. Nancy thought this was a great idea, and we headed off for Nantucket. It was late in the tourist season so the island wasn't crowded. We spent a romantic day walking on the beach and looking at quaint stores. We had a candlelight supper at one of the island's best restaurants. And then we went back to the inn and made love. This time it took more stimulation to get an erection, but I really wasn't as hard as I had always been in the past, and I lost my erection quickly.

When we got back from the island, I really started to worry. I "knew" there wasn't anything wrong with me psychologically. I felt very confident about that. I was tremendously attracted to Nancy. I started to think that there might be a physical problem and that I should go see a doctor. But that thought frightened me. They say that people in the health professions take terrible care of themselves. That's not a myth. As a lab technician who worked in a hospital, I knew there were plenty of serious physical problems that could be causing me to be impotent . . . and I just didn't want to think about them. So I shrugged off doing anything for a while.

I continued to see Nancy because I liked her so much, but now I found myself manipulating her so that we wouldn't get into sexual situations. I'd use the old routines women once used on me: "Darling, not now, I've got a headache" or "I don't feel well" or "Let's watch a good movie on TV." Nancy went along with this for a while.

Until one night, when my passions got the better of me. We were lying in front of Nancy's fireplace, cuddling, listening to some romantic music — it was straight out of the worst grade-B movie. We just tore at each other. But nothing happened. It was humiliating.

I don't think I've ever been so embarrassed in my entire life. I was standing there with no clothes on, she was standing there with no clothes on. We just started at each other. I couldn't get an erection. I was semihard, but nothing you could penetrate with, nothing you could be proud of. I'd never felt so embarrassed in front of a woman before. And the way Nancy looked at me — it was almost like she was looking at me and I wasn't there. Or maybe she *wished* I wasn't there.

SEEKING TREATMENT

As amazing as it seems now, we tried to make love at least a half dozen times after the incident in front of the fireplace. Each time was the same. Finally, I told Nancy that I was going to go see Dr. Irwin Goldstein, a urologist who I had heard worked in the area of impotence.

When I went to see Dr. Goldstein, he did an ultrasound study to check the blood flow to my penis. [*Ultrasonography* uses high-frequency sound waves to measure blood flow (see box, page 77).] I checked out all right, although the blood pressure in my penis was slightly lower than normal.

Then he gave me a test in which I slipped little electrodes over my penis that recorded any changes in its circumference during the night — that was supposed to indicate whether I had erections while I was sleeping, as men normally do. The test demonstrated reasonable amounts of circumference changes during the night erections.

Dr. Goldstein recommended that I see a psychologist, but I refused. A couple of months went by, and Nancy started to put pressure on me to see the therapist that Dr. Goldstein had recommended. We were still seeing each other, but Nancy told me that I was changing. She said that I was becoming less patient, less tolerant and less sociable. I didn't want to go out with friends or do anything. Sometimes friends would come over and we'd have a few drinks, and someone would tell a joke involving sex. Once, after such a party, Nancy told me, "You should have seen your expression. Right away you became quiet as if the joke was about you. You were gone," she said, "and I knew you were gone." I had never been conscious of my reactions until she told me about them.

Nancy kept after me to see a therapist, or at least to talk to her about what I was feeling. But I wouldn't. I was keeping it all to myself. I was thinking: What is wrong with me? Am I changing? You think of everything.

I even thought, maybe it's Nancy. Maybe I'm not attracted to her. But after all the years of being divorced and going out with women, I felt I'd finally found that person I should have found many years before. I was attracted to her, and I enjoyed just sitting with her and talking about life, or about any subject at all. I was comfortable with her.

That's what made it so difficult—it was a great relationship. If we had limited ourselves to seeing each other on weekends, maybe things would have been easier on both of us. But we enjoyed each other so much. When I got out of work, we'd get the kids and go down to the beach, go out to eat or just go for a walk together. We were so happy except when it came time to make love.

All during this time, we continued to try to have sex. That really made things terrible. I still had desire. I was like a volcano. I wanted to erupt. But nothing. Nothing.

Over and over again, nothing. And I kept playing this game inside my head. Just like when your car doesn't start. You always say, maybe next time. That's how I felt. Every time I tried and failed, I'd say maybe next time. But nothing ever happened. And I couldn't call a medical AAA to come over and jump-start me. So our repeated efforts just led to more and more frustration for me and for Nancy.

Nancy was going through hell during this time. She'd break down crying almost every night. She thought it was her problem, that my impotence was caused by her inability to stimulate me enough.

Nancy knew my past history, she knew that I'd had a lot of sexual experience with women. So she automatically assumed, "Well, he's been fine all these years and all of a sudden he's going out with me and he can't perform. It's got to be me." I knew that wasn't true and I tried to console her, telling her it was my ineptness that was the problem. But after so many failures, I got to the point where I just couldn't cope with it all anymore. I decided to go back to see Dr. Goldstein, hoping maybe something would show up this time.

Dr. Goldstein decided to do an arteriogram. [An *arteriogram* is an X-ray picture of the arteries in the groin and in the penis (see box, page 78).] If there was blockage, then that was the cause of my impotence. The test showed that the blood vessels just outside my penis and inside my penis were very small. Dr. Goldstein was quite suspicious that this was my problem—arterial blockage—but he still wanted me to see the sex therapist. He wasn't sure an operation could fix the problem.

HOPE AND DESPAIR

Now I'm thinking: Is this really *in my head*? Why is this happening to me?

After the arteriogram, I was such a wreck that I decided to take a couple of weeks off. I rented a house on the Cape and took Nancy and the kids. We had a great time. And we tried again sexually. After lots of foreplay and lots of concentration, on the last night, I finally got a good erection that lasted and lasted. We had sex for hours. I felt alive for the first time in months. It was amazing. Nancy is shouting "Wooooow! This is great! Where has this been all these months!" And I'm thinking, "I'm better. I don't believe this! I'm better."

That was the last time we had sex for seven months. I never got another erection, no matter what we tried. Later, Dr. Goldstein explained to me that with my type of partial arterial blockage, I was able to get a good erection (but still not a "normal" one) only with continuous, prolonged stimulation under ideal conditions—like being on vacation. But, at the time, this one success in the midst of continued failure seemed a special torture.

My life had never been so terrible. I started to miss work, pretending to be sick. I started drinking a lot, spending a lot of my time at the sports bar. I didn't care if the world caved in. I just couldn't deal with my problems anymore. After a few drinks, my troubles would go away and I thought of more pleasant things.

I didn't see Nancy that much during this time. I couldn't handle it. I felt embarrassed when I was around her, even though we still enjoyed each other. Also, I knew she still wanted me to see a psychologist. And I still didn't want to. Looking back, I think I was afraid the therapist was going to tell me I was crazy. I felt so crazy all the time, but being told I was really crazy was the one thing I knew I couldn't deal with.

I did end up going to the therapist Dr. Goldstein recommended. But it wasn't because of Nancy's urging. As strange as it seems, my ex-wife Carol was the one who got through to me. She wouldn't let me see Tom, Jr. on weekends anymore. Carol told me that she didn't know what was the matter with me, but Tom, Jr. had told her about my drinking and my general state of unhappiness. She didn't want to put Tom, Jr. through any more grief.

That really struck home. Being a father, a good father, was what had held me together when I went through my divorce. Just knowing my son was there and that I wanted him to have a good life had sustained me. I had wanted him to know that he had a father who really loved him, no matter what the problems were between his mother and me. Now, it seemed, even that cherished relationship was being threatened by my "problem."

My therapist, Dr. Alma Dell Smith, explained that I was in a "reactive depression," that I'd experienced a loss — my potency — and I was reacting to it, just as if someone I'd loved had died. Interestingly, I was going through the same stages that people go through when someone is dying — denial, anger, bargaining with God and grief.

So the problem wasn't my impotence, but the way I was *reacting* to it. Underlying everything, the therapist told me, was the fact that I still couldn't accept that my impotence didn't have a physical cause. She urged me to go back to see Dr. Goldstein.

A DIAGNOSIS AND A TREATMENT PLAN

Dr. Goldstein decided to do a second, more extensive sleep test that required me to stay in the hospital for two nights. In addition to monitoring the circumference changes of my penis, they photographed my erection and determined how rigid the erection was by putting a weight on the head of the penis during an erection. I didn't have the normal rigidity in the erections in my sleep either night even though I had relatively normal circumference changes.

Now Dr. Goldstein confirmed that there was something physically wrong down there. I really felt for the first time as if a tremendous burden had been lifted. I knew I was impotent, physiologically impotent. What once would have brought instant terror to me, now was the best news of my life. It was great for Nancy also. Finally her burden of not being able to arouse me was lifted.

Dr. Goldstein explained that there were different approaches to handling my problem — now defined as physical impotence most likely due to partial arterial blockage, or "failure to fill": I could have a penile implant; I could undergo revascularization surgery to take care of the blockage in my arteries; I could continue with sex therapy to reduce anxiety; or I could go on a drug program using papaverine, which is injected into the penis to relax its smooth-muscle tissue. I decided on the injections. [In 1983, *papaverine* was introduced as a treatment for impotence. These days, we more commonly use a combination of drugs, including *papaverine, phentolamine* and sometimes *prostaglandin E1* because combinations of drugs appear to be more effective than individual drugs in treating impotence (see chapter 6 for more information about penile injections).]

I came to Dr. Goldstein's office and he injected me. I got a slowly developing erection, but one that was ultimately reasonably rigid.

Dr. Goldstein told me it could possibly be good for a couple of hours. I rushed out to call Nancy. I told her, "I just had my first shot, I'm coming up to see you, just get ready." So I jumped into my car and started on the expressway and I lost my erection. It hadn't been more than fifty minutes since the injection.

I couldn't believe it. All I could think was, why? Why? What have I done to deserve this? What the hell have I done? I was so distraught I pulled off the road and started to cry.

After that, Dr. Goldstein decided to teach me to perform the injections myself. I'll tell you, you have to be close to your limit to want to inject your penis with something.

The first time, I really had to work up the nerve to go and do it. I was thinking, "Tom, you've done some pretty crazy things in your life, and now you're sticking a needle in your penis. This has to be the craziest!" But even though it was crazy, I had to do it. I had to get that erection. But still nothing. Nothing. I would get semihard, but that was all. Dr. Goldstein suggested that he perform surgery for the suspected arterial blockages. After talking with Nancy, I decided to go ahead. That was in September.

SURGERY

I had the surgery in December. For six weeks after the surgery, Nancy and I were told not to have sex. Dr. Goldstein wanted to make sure that those vessels stayed sewed together. I didn't get an erection until about twelve days after the surgery. And all during this period, running through my mind is the question: Is this going to work? After all I'd been through, I really didn't think anything was going to happen.

But now, here's a funny thing. There are so many paradoxes about impotence. You want an erection. You dream about it, think about it all the time. But the first erection after the operation—I was praying for the damned thing to go away. I was in excruciating pain. It was eleven o'clock in the morning, I remember. A Friday morning. I was watching television, an old rerun of the "Andy Griffith Show," when lo and behold, I got an erection. For no reason at all, all of a sudden I felt that warm flow. I ran into the bathroom and looked in the mirror—Wooooow! There it was! It looked extremely large to me because it had been so long since I'd seen it. I didn't know if it was me.

But then, all of a sudden, it started throbbing. I was afraid to touch it. It was killing me until finally it went down. And that's the way it was for the next six weeks. I'd get up in the middle of the night with an erection—it would wake me right up, it would be so painful—and I would double up. I'd groan, "Go away, go away." It was just incredible pain. But after a few weeks, things started to normalize and the pain went away.

Nancy and I started to have sex. The first time was incredible. We made love for hours. And we both cried, but this time for joy. I always enjoyed sex, but I used to take it for granted, like breathing. But now that I could perform again after being impotent, I savored every moment. Nancy said, "So this is why your friends called you Tom the Lover." And I told her, "Honestly, this is better."

CONFIDENCE

I have incredible confidence now, more than I ever had before. I feel like I could deal with any crisis. I'd had crises in my life before—my divorce was terrible—but not like this. This was something I had to overcome and deal with all by myself. It taught me to be stronger than I ever thought I could be. Stronger emotionally. More self-reliant.

Ten months after the operation, Nancy and I got married. Some of my friends have asked me if Nancy and I would have married if I had still been impotent. My answer is, "Hell, no." How could have I tied her down with a man who couldn't make love to her? She was only thirty-two. No, I couldn't have asked her, no matter how much I loved her. I couldn't do the things that a woman expects of a man. From the time they're born, men are told that sexual abilities are very important in life. Whether it's true or not, that's the thought in your mind. When you lose your potency, as I did, you can lose all your self-esteem.

I'm somebody who enjoys being with women, enjoys the pleasure I get with women. And I was in a relationship with somebody I really cared about. If you can't function sexually, you feel you're "not human." I know it's wrong to feel that way, but that's how I felt.

I think it's the same for some people when they lose a job. There's this feeling of being lost. I can't explain it fully. I felt empty. It was like there was somebody else in there screaming to get out, looking for the Tom that used to be and was no longer. It was draining, completely draining, especially because I felt I couldn't talk about it with anyone. When you have friends, family, your ex-wife, asking you what's wrong with you, how do you explain to them? How do you tell them, "I'm impotent"?

I couldn't tell anybody. My worst mistake was that I held my feelings in too long. I thought: I'm a man. I can handle this. I don't need help. But that's foolishness. So what if you bend people's ears? Bend their ears. That's what people are for. A friend, a priest, anybody. You've got to let that feeling out. You get to a point where you want everybody to know. I wanted the whole world to know. I got so tired of keeping it in. And I want women to understand, if they've got a boyfriend or a husband with this problem, what that emptiness feels like. Men should feel that they can be helped, that they can get back their life just as I did.

Dr. Irwin Goldstein:
The Medical Perspective

Tom came to the clinic for evaluation in February 1984. His experience reflects our state of medical knowledge at that time, and serves as a reminder of how quickly our knowledge is evolving. Were Tom to walk into the clinic today, he would receive a battery of tests unavailable back in 1984. Prominent among them would be *DICC* studies—short for "dynamic infusion cavernosometry and cavernosography" (see box, page 102). DICC studies are erection chamber and blood-pressure measurements as well as X rays of the penis's storage system taken during a state of erection. Arteriograms (see box, page 78) enable us to look at arteries. DICC studies enable us also to look at veins and to get information about the penis's erectile tissue. Tom's story remains significant, however, because he helped demonstrate that certain surgical procedures could correct impotence caused by arterial blockage.

During his first appointment in early 1984, Tom impressed me as an anxious, somewhat angry and frustrated young man. He answered my questions about his medical history with short, snappish answers, one foot tapping in agitation on the floor. With a few notable exceptions, he had been impotent for the last nine months. His emotional state was not unusual—it simply reflected how devastating a sudden, unexpected sexual dysfunction can be, especially for an otherwise healthy young man.

INJURIES

I learned that he had been in two accidents that involved his pelvis—one when he was a twelve-year-old, riding his bicycle, and a second fourteen years later, on his motorcycle. Although neither accident had been major, both delivered solid knocks to his perineum, where the internal portion of his penis was located. Perineal injuries should sound an alarm in a urologist's mind because *blunt perineal trauma,* injury to the perineal area (see illustration, page 76), may figure in the origins of a man's impotence. I'd say it probably did in Tom's case based on the evidence we obtained later from his arteriogram.

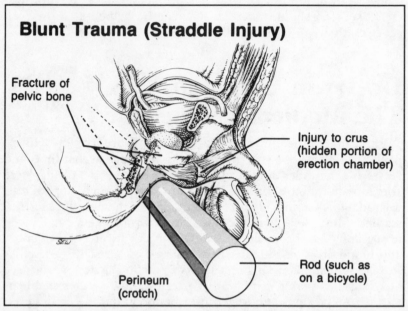

Blunt Trauma (Straddle Injury)

Fracture of
pelvic bone

Injury to crus
(hidden portion of
erection chamber)

Perineum
(crotch)

Rod (such as
on a bicycle)

In this example of blunt trauma, a rod is striking the pelvis and perineum in a straddle accident, resulting in a pelvic fracture and injury to the perineum. Blunt injury to the pelvis or perineum (with or without pelvic fracture) may result in injury to the arteries supplying blood to the erection chambers and cause "failure to fill." Blunt perineal trauma may also injure the hidden portions of the erection chambers, the right and left crura, which may result in erection-tissue scarring and "failure to store" in this part of the penis.

BLOOD PRESSURE

After the history and physical examination, the next logical step was to do an ultrasound check of the blood pressure in Tom's penis (see box, page 77).

In Tom's case, we found the pressure in his penis was only 75 percent of the pressure in his arm. What did this mean? By itself, any symptom or test result may be inconclusive, but in combination with other observations, the result may be indicative of a particular problem. Tom's penile blood-pressure readings were somewhat low, but not alarmingly so. In light of his accidents, I suspected that the circulation in his penis was impaired. But I needed additional evidence before I could make a solid diagnosis.

NOCTURNAL ERECTIONS

I asked Tom to keep track of his nocturnal (nighttime) erections with a portable monitor. The monitor was wired to a soft mercury-

Penile Doppler Ultrasound

Ultrasonography has become familiar to the public as a convenient, painless way for expectant parents to get their first glimpse of the developing fetus. Another application is its use as a stethoscope, for taking blood pressures, such as in the penis.

The newest application of penile ultrasound is duplex Doppler ultrasound. In this examination, the ultrasound waves are able to examine the consistency of the erection tissue and the lining of the erection chamber, the tunica. The ultrasound is also able to localize each of the two erection arteries, record their individual diameter and measure the velocity of blood flow through each artery. The study is best performed in the erect state after injection of erection-producing drugs into the side of the base of the penis via a small insulin needle. Men who have small diameter artery blood vessels with reduced velocity of blood flow during erection may have an artery blockage or a "failure to fill" erection problem. Blockages in the arteries that deliver blood to the erection chambers during erection will also cause reduced pressure in the cavernosal (erection) arteries. A direct recording of the pressure in the erection arteries, which can be simultaneously compared to the pressure of the arteries in the arm (they should be the same) may be measured during a DICC study (see box, page 102)

filled ring, which Tom slipped over his penis before retiring at night. If the circumference of his penis changed while Tom slept, indicating an erection, it would be recorded by the monitor. Known as a *Nocturnal Penile Tumescence Test*, the study is run for two consecutive nights; it records whether a patient is getting erections and, if so, how often. A normal pattern of nocturnal erectile activity (most men have an average of four erections per night) often suggests a psychological origin for impotence, whereas an abnormal pattern of changes may reflect a physical problem.

This test demonstrated that there were reasonable circumference changes in Tom's penis associated with the nighttime erections. Unfortunately, circumference changes do not reliably reflect the rigidity of the erection. In other words, Tom could have reasonable circumference changes but still have inadequate rigidity in his erections.

I decided to do more tests, including an arteriogram (see box, below). The arteriogram showed that the arteries in Tom's flaccid penis, as well as the arteries leading to it, were suspiciously narrow. I doubted that enough blood was getting through these arteries to give Tom normal erections. (Nowadays, we are doing arteriograms on erect penises, but in early 1984 we were only able to study the penis's arteries in the flaccid state.)

The Arteriogram

An *arteriogram* is an X ray of the arteries leading to, and inside, the penis. In early 1984 we were only performing arteriograms of flaccid penises. At the present time we perform such studies in the erect state under sedation with greater ability to observe the arteries in the penis for the presence of any blockages.

The arteriogram is performed in the X-ray department by a radiologist. An anesthetic solution, *novocaine*, is injected into the skin of the patient's groin. The doctor then introduces a small-diameter tube (about the size of the tip of a ballpoint pen) through the anesthetized skin into an artery of the leg. While the doctor is watching an X-ray screen, he or she is able to enter virtually any artery in the body from the leg artery. In this particular study, the artery to the erection chamber is studied during a drug-induced erection.

An arteriogram is the most sophisticated study available in impotence diagnosis. At Boston University Medical Center, it is presently performed on those patients who wish to consider vascular reconstructive surgery and who, after a DICC study, demonstrate low blood pressure in the erection artery as well as an absence of multiple blood-storage problems. In our clinic, we recommend arteriograms for only five to ten out of every 100 patients being evaluated for impotence.

FAILURE TO FILL

In terms of the discussion in chapter 2, Tom was experiencing a "failure to fill" (see page 27).

I can now look at Tom's medical record and deduce that his erectile system probably had a good blood-storage mechanism. In 1984, we had not yet learned about the storage mechanism, or learned to appreciate the role it plays in erectile physiology. The fact that Tom could occasionally achieve a rigid erection for a sustained time leads me to conclude, in retrospect, that he was one of those relatively rare patients—about 20 percent of impotent patients—with blocked arteries and a filling problem who did *not* also have problems with blood storage. Approximately 80 percent of the patients in my practice with arterial blockage also have difficulty with blood storage within the erect penis.

Tom's particular type of impotence—blocked arteries, in combination with an effective storage mechanism—is very difficult to diagnose, even today, with our improved ability to measure such things.

I often explain this type of impotence to men by asking them to imagine two neighbors, each of whom owns a swimming pool. A swimming pool, like the penis, has an effective storage system. Once you fill it with water, the water won't leak out.

But how will each fill it?

Let's assume each neighbor has his own way of filling his pool. The first neighbor uses an ordinary garden hose. He rises at dawn, starts the water flowing, and then waits all day as the pool slowly fills. By the early evening the pool is filled, and he's able to take his first swim of the season.

This was how Tom's penis behaved. His storage mechanism, like the pool's, was excellent, but his ability to fill, like that of the garden hose, was very slow. With no external stresses—during vacations, for example, with the whole day for making love—Tom's penis would eventually become erect. But once he returned to civilization, with all its hassles, he didn't have time to wait for his slow-filling penis to get an erection, and his vulnerability to psychological factors slowed his filling even more.

Now let's look at the second neighbor. He returns home from a long day on the job, feeling run-down and irritated. Then he has an inspiration: How about a swim? As a member of the local volunteer fire department, he borrows a wide-bore fire hose and attaches it to the hydrant in front of his house. Water blasts into his pool, filling it in a short period of time. How exciting! One minute he's hot and tired; a short while later he's enjoying a refreshing dip.

The second neighbor's pool is analogous to a man whose penis has a good storage mechanism and has healthy arteries, ready to deliver a rich supply of blood to his erection at a moment's notice. A healthy man's erections are spontaneous, quick to develop, and rigid, but a man with compromised penile arteries usually experiences slow-developing, partial erections.

A PSYCHOLOGICAL COMPONENT

This type of impotence also frequently features a secondary psychological component, and in fact is often misdiagnosed as psychogenic impotence. The man's primary problem is indeed physical, but his secondary psychological reactions to it compound the dysfunction.

Tom's mood during our interviews clearly indicated that his erectile problems were taking a toll on his emotions. After the inconclusive results of Tom's initial tests, I suggested he see a therapist. He was evaluated by Dr. Smith, but he declined further therapy. In certain respects Tom was a casualty of the type of outdated thinking that is still pervasive among many men. He was terrified of psychological therapy; a therapist might confirm his worst fear, that his impotence was psychological, that he was "going crazy." Ironically, these fears themselves may have had a very definite effect on his erectile ability.

AN AGING ERECTILE SYSTEM

Over the course of a man's life, his erections become *increasingly vulnerable to the influence of psychological factors*. It's easy to understand why this should be by looking at how his erectile physiology changes as a man ages (see box, page 25).

As a young adult, his erectile tissue is highly elastic; his storage mechanism is effective; the arteries to his penis are unobstructed, and a rich supply of blood reaches his erectile tissue. He can achieve a rigid erection lasting fifteen to twenty minutes. Psychological conflicts, even if present, often lack the power to override his powerful erectile physiology.

But if you add thirty or forty years to his age, what happens? All of those factors I just mentioned are in decline: His erectile tissue may be less elastic; smoking and overindulgence in fatty food may have taken their toll on his smooth-muscle tissue; he may have an arterial blockage or two. When men reach their fifties and sixties, they commonly experience erections sufficient for intercourse, but the fact is, they often have some physical impairment that reduces their function to 60 to 80 percent of their previous capabilities. In their compromised state, the influence of psychological factors on their performance becomes much stronger.

Tom was only thirty-nine, but he already had a decreased supply of blood to his erectile tissue. Under these conditions, the effects of anxiety and worry may have made the situation worse by undermining the ability of his smooth-muscle tissue to relax. Without this relaxation, the flow of blood was further restricted and the lacunar spaces in his erection chambers couldn't fill with blood. In short, he couldn't become erect.

ARTERIAL BLOCKAGE: OPTIONS FOR CURE

In May of 1984, four months after Tom's first visit to my office, he spent a couple of nights in the hospital undergoing a more extensive record of his nocturnal erections and measuring the rigidity of the night erections. The test further confirmed that Tom had abnormal erections and indicated a probable impairment in Tom's circulation.

I told Tom his impotence was probably primarily physical — not primarily psychological. It was possible that his arteries had been injured in his two accidents. The *endothelium*, a lining of specialized cells that covers the inner surface of the arteries (see illustration, page 13), is especially susceptible in an accident; the compression of an artery between the pelvic bone and a bicycle seat, for instance, can permanently damage the circulation (see illustration, page 76).

Research has shown that places where the endothelium is injured often become the site of an arterial blockage. Tom's bicycle accident happened many years ago, but it's probable that injuries to his endothelium became the focus for his subsequent blockages.

I offered Tom four options — sex therapy to reduce his anxiety, papaverine injections to dilate the penile vessels, revascularization surgery to improve blood flow to the penis or a penile implant to give him dependable, but "artificial," erections.

SEX THERAPY

Sex therapy may not seem like a logical response to organic impotence, but I want to stress that a diagnosis of organic impotence does not mean that a patient *must* have it corrected. For some men and their partners, reassurance that their problem is indeed physical, rather than psychological, is satisfactory medical intervention, and therapy can help them adjust to their diminished potency. This is often true in elderly men, who neither wish to have injections nor undergo surgery. Although Tom was still young, had he not chosen one of the other treatments, sex therapy could have helped him and Nancy maintain their sexual intimacy with less emphasis on intercourse. Although they did not have sex therapy, Tom did have an evaluation visit with Dr. Alma Dell Smith.

REVASCULARIZATION SURGERY

Revascularization, a surgical procedure, also called *arterial bypass* surgery, would increase the flow of blood to his penis by bypassing

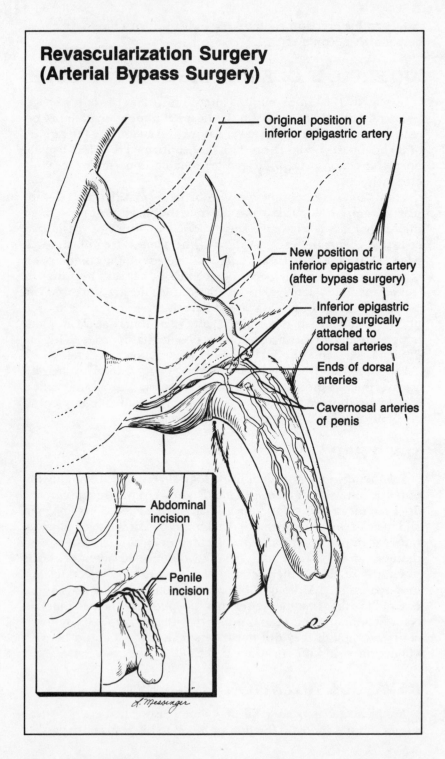

Revascularization Surgery (Arterial Bypass Surgery)

Original position of inferior epigastric artery

New position of inferior epigastric artery (after bypass surgery)

Inferior epigastric artery surgically attached to dorsal arteries

Ends of dorsal arteries

Cavernosal arteries of penis

Abdominal incision

Penile incision

L. Messinger

the blocked portions of his arteries. The procedure would then recon-
nect the arteries to normal blood vessels, capable of accepting the
new blood flow (see illustration, page 82).

The drawback to this procedure was that Tom's arteriogram on
his flaccid penis failed to show *any* normal arteries in his penis. It
didn't follow that all his penile arteries were necessarily too narrow,
but we wouldn't know for sure until after we had operated. Since
the arteriogram didn't enable me to predict a successful surgical outcome, the bypass option wasn't clear-cut.

Tom wanted to think about his choices before making any decisions. For the next several months his treatment was suspended.

PAPAVERINE INJECTIONS

Tom returned to the office in August of 1984, resolved to initially
try papaverine treatment. *Papaverine,* a chemical that can be injected
into the penis, relaxes the smooth-muscle tissue of the corpora cavernosa to encourage the development of an erection. (I'll say more
about injections in chapter 6. Papaverine is seldom used alone in
penile injections nowadays.) His first injection, as he points out in
his narrative, didn't last as long as he would have liked. My guess
is that he was somewhat anxious so that his nervous tension ultimately
overrode the effect of the injection. Subsequent home self-injection
therapy wasn't successful either. In October, after talking it over with
his girlfriend, he decided to try revascularization.

THE SURGERY

By the time of Tom's surgery in December of 1984, I'd had three
years of experience with revascularization surgery. At the present
time, I have performed over 350 such procedures. I'd first begun performing this kind of surgery in 1981, several months after a visit
to Boston by the father of vascular reconstructive surgery, Dr. Vaclav
Michal of Czechoslovakia. He had performed the first arterial
reconstructions for impotence in 1973. There was a flurry of interest
in the United States in the early seventies, but it ended quickly when
the first American patients failed to do well.

Today, physicians are becoming increasingly convinced of the value
of vascular surgery for impotence treatment in well-selected,

---

"Failure-to-fill" erection insufficiency can sometimes be treated with revascularization surgery, in which the artery blockage is bypassed using a leg artery
branch called the inferior epigastric artery. This artery may be surgically attached
to the dorsal arteries of the penis. Higher blood pressure and increased blood
flow to the penis may be achieved with this surgery.

specific circumstances. But, in science, as in life, first impressions mean a lot.

In the earliest version of the operation, the bypass artery was connected directly to the erectile tissue for which the blood was destined. But within a short time the arterial connections to the erectile tissue became blocked and the erectile capacity of these patients failed to improve. A later version of the operation would correctly connect the bypass artery to a second healthy artery leading to the erectile tissue, rather than directly to the tissue itself (see illustration, page 82). Nevertheless, revascularization surgery (arterial bypass surgery) for impotence was labeled unpredictable, experimental and short-term.

Interest centered mainly around penile implants for many years. Despite problems, especially with the early models, implants demonstrated more reliable long-term success in the treatment of impotence. Personally, I prefer to regard an implant as the treatment of last resort because its installation irreversibly damages the erectile tissue. Innovations in vascular surgery are constantly broadening the spectrum of patients whose own erectile physiology can be restored. But for a man with an implant, there's no going back— he's committed. In an elderly man, this may not be a problem, but for a young man, why close the door on the possibility of fixing his problem in the future?

Tom was in surgery for eight hours. Fortunately, it turned out the arteries in the penis we couldn't see on his arteriogram were indeed there and were intact. We rerouted an artery from his abdominal wall and connected it to two arteries in his penis. Tom was in the hospital for three days, recuperated several weeks at home and within two weeks of the surgery was getting good erections.

A NORMAL SEX LIFE

Soon Tom was able to resume a normal sex life. Ten months after the operation, he and Nancy were married and they now have a child. His erections remain strong now, five years later. When I performed the operation we thought that the results would be long-term but there was no patient data to support my conviction. Numerous studies since Tom's case have confirmed the effectiveness of revascularization surgery in similar kinds of situations—where the patient has only a few, well-defined arterial blockages. At present, urologists are much more capable of predicting which reconstructive cases will be successful than they were at the time of Tom's surgery, especially with diagnostic testing of the storage mechanism, which was not widely utilized back in 1984.

Dr. Alma Dell Smith—
The Psychological Perspective

I saw Tom Killian for an evaluation session and was given permission to review his case history and taped interviews.

It goes without saying that a man's identity is based partly on his sexual identity. Tom's expertise as a lover was a major part of his identity. Because sex figured so prominently in his image of himself, his reaction to his impotence was magnified. Tom says he experienced a profound sense of loss when he became impotent.

For many men, like Tom, impotence involves a significant decline in their pride in being a man. A man feels a surprising degree of shame when he can't get an erection, as if it were somehow his fault, a crime he committed against the world. Given the extent to which men congratulate themselves for simply functioning normally, maybe it's to be expected that they also feel responsible for *failing* to function normally. "If we're going to take the credit," so the reasoning goes, "we should also take the blame when things don't work as they should."

But the losses involved in impotence go far beyond the loss of pride. As Tom suggests, the loss of potency can plunge a man into despair. Sexual functioning is how we live—if we don't procreate, as a species, we simply don't survive on this planet—and some form of that message is programmed into every cell of our bodies. So it is not exaggerating to say that when you discover you can't function sexually anymore, you can almost feel "not human," as Tom described.

For Tom, this feeling was exaggerated when what he thought his private dilemma became something others could see as well. To have his friends say, "Tom, what's wrong?" when he hadn't said anything was wrong, to have his ex-wife say, "I don't think you ought to see Tom, Jr. for a while," when Tom, Jr. was the person who stood between him and suicide, forced Tom to come face-to-face with the fact that his personality was crumbling. Not only in his own eyes, but in everybody else's too. Tom, in his mind, had not only lost his potency, but he felt he had actually lost himself.

Loss is extremely difficult for most men to deal with. It demands the acknowledgment of such "unmasculine" traits as dependency and vulnerability, and it involves a constantly changing mix of profound and conflicting feelings. Untrained as men are in our culture to become acquainted with their emotions and to learn how to manage them without repressing them, they often find the flood of feelings involved with loss to be overwhelming. We see it in men who have lost their wives. We see it in men who have lost a child.

We see it in men who have lost their jobs. They don't know how to cope with loss.

But when the loss to be grieved is a crucial and integral part of the self, the problem becomes more complex. It is not unusual, for instance, when a man has lost his wife for him to feel that somehow he has died. But eventually there comes a recognition that his wife was a separate entity from him, and that while she has died, he lives on.

The loss of potency is much more insidious than that—and because of that, it can be harder to handle. It is a fundamental part of yourself that has "died." You are not a separate entity from it.

If you have lost your potency, whether you understand why or not, it is important to realize that all the feelings you are experiencing are absolutely to be expected, and that they do not mean that you are also losing your mind. You have every right to be angry, to feel afraid and to get so frustrated you think you're going to explode. Sex is one of the three most powerful forces driving us from within—along with hunger and thirst—and if it can't find expression, the pressure that builds behind it is enough to make anyone think he is losing his mind.

DEFUSING ANXIETY

It is important to realize that if you don't do something with those feelings, you just *may* go out of your mind. If your feelings aren't expressed and released, they will create pressures in you that have to make room for themselves. In order to make room for themselves, they have to shift things around in you—that's why Tom's personality changed when he became impotent.

Obviously, you're not going to go around with a name tag saying, "Hi! My name is Tom and I'm impotent!" But if you can't talk about this problem with the people who matter to you, you may not ever be able to relax the smooth-muscle tissue of the penis enough to function normally again. *It is part of the nature of impotence that once it begins, it builds on itself because the anxiety it provokes actually makes the problem worse.*

Somewhere the circle has to be broken. Most men find that talking about their impotence helps to defuse their anxiety. And if you find it difficult or pointless to talk to family or friends, there are several organizations designed to bring men together to work on their shared problems (see the list of support groups at the back of this book).

A HAPPY ENDING

It is a measure of Tom's psychological health that he recognized the depth of his problem and got himself the help that he needed.

He was certainly reluctant, but he brought himself around and that was the start of the end of the problem.

Another thing that pulled Tom through was that his confidence in himself and in his sexual functioning was basically strong and only superficially shaken by his impotence. Even when his self-confidence began to erode, there remained a knot of conviction somewhere deep inside of him that he was mentally OK. When it was finally determined that there was a physiological cause to his impotence, his confidence was ready for service. His faith in himself and his sexuality returned quickly.

Not everyone is that lucky. Tom seems to be blessed with a relatively uncomplicated psyche. But if a man's personality is more complex and intricate, the effects of impotence may feed into other insecurities and undermine his sense of himself in a more profound way. If a man has always secretly felt that there was "something wrong" with him, especially if that something involves his sexuality, then impotence is all the evidence necessary for him to "prove" his own lack of self-worth. In other chapters we'll describe men who follow this pattern.

For Tom, the story had a happy ending. He is married again, a father again, a lover of life again.

CHAPTER 5

David–
A Tale of Two Surgeries

The patient in this chapter, David Herzog (not his real name), came to our impotence clinic in 1987, some three years after Tom Killian, the patient in chapter 4. At the time, he was thirty-eight years old, married and employed as a university botanist. David's arterial blockages and his defective blood-storage mechanism caused him to have an erectile insufficiency. Two surgeries, one involving both revascularization *(see chapter 4) and* venous ligation, *and the other involving* crural plication, *restored his potency.* Venous ligation *is the tying off of veins.* Crural plication *tightens the* tunica albuginea *in the hidden portion of the penis. These latter procedures are vascular reconstructive procedures designed to increase the resistance to blood drainage during an erection and thus treat "failure-to-store" erection problems. While significant advances have been made in these surgical procedures in the last several years, follow-up has revealed poor long-term success rates.*

David's Story

My wife Becky and I had more than our share of turmoil in the early years of our relationship. Some of this was beyond our control, the consequence of our decision to emigrate from Israel and the stress of scrambling around the world so I could finish my graduate degree in botany. As long as we've known each other, we've had to struggle with our sexual relationship.

My wife and I first met in 1976. She was twenty-seven; I was twenty-six. We were working in the botany department of the University of Jerusalem. She was intensely attracted to me, but I hardly knew who she was. She was the equivalent of what's called an assistant professor in the United States. I was a graduate student, but we hadn't come across each other.

She was leading a field course for undergraduates, and as one of the eight graduate students, I was expected to go and listen to this course, partly to brush up on my lichens (plants that grow on solid surfaces), and also to get some experience in handling students. I went reluctantly, because I wasn't really interested in lichens. If it grew on a rock, I wasn't interested in it.

I was put into her group and I admit I liked her. We talked a lot about work. Becky's low-key—I like that—but I could tell that she was incredibly bright. She was also beautiful. The week went by, we had quite a lot of fun and we sort of saw each other afterwards. Then I noticed that she kept coming into the lab where I was working. As graduate students, we had a lab to ourselves, but for some reason Becky had suddenly had all sorts of excuses to come in.

Suddenly it dawned on me—she was attracted to me. I felt the same way about her, but I resisted my feelings. I tried to push my feelings aside. This friend of mine, a woman named Michelle, had died in February, and it had been so traumatic I had decided to put all my attention on my work. I couldn't afford to do badly, so I didn't want to get involved with anybody.

I tried to ignore Becky, but these were very strong feelings. I remember borrowing a pair of binoculars from her for a bird-watching assignment, and then going to return them on a Sunday afternoon. It finally registered that we were nuts about each other. The first thing she wanted to do was to have sex.

We sat out on her balcony and we were just crazy about each other. She really wanted to go and jump straight in the sack right then and there, but she said, "Well, maybe I shouldn't, because I'm not taking the pill and I think I'm ovulating, so we'd better be careful."

So we decided we would wait a few weeks. We saw each other a lot over the next two weeks. Days and nights, a whole week would go by, and I hadn't done my laundry. It was so incredibly intense, the time seemed to be all contracted.

When we finally did go to bed, it was a bust. She was pretty disappointed, and, of course, so was I. I didn't know how to deal with it. I don't know if she said it then or the time after that, but she said, "Well, are you sure you're not gay?" That made me twist and turn inside.

From the very beginning things went awry. We would have sex and it wouldn't work, and then we'd say, "Well, OK, what's going on?" We soon realized that each of us was trying to figure out if something the other person was doing was somehow sabotaging our lovemaking. Well, you know you can't blame the other person. Then

I'd say, "Well, now what's the matter? Is it because I'm exhausted?" We hassled with it for months.

The year finished and I got my graduate degree. I was going to do military service, but first we went away for a week and we had a wonderful time. We had reasonably good sex and everything seemed fine. I then went into military training. We didn't see each other for about two or three months at all and then we'd see other sporadically, but somehow the relationship seemed OK. Not great, but OK.

STRESS

As long as I was in the military we kept attributing the difficulties to my stresses connected to where I was stationed. The following year in April we decided to live together. Once again we saw that there was something weird going on in our sexual relationship. During vacations, if I relaxed enough, and if she relaxed enough, then our sexual relationship would seem fine. So it didn't seem that there was that much of a problem. That was our pattern.

We decided that I was impotent from the stress and pressure. That became our rationale for years, because God knows, we did have more than the usual share of stress in our lives—the trauma of leaving Israel and all that.

We married and then traveled through Europe for six months. We did some work in southern France, living in the back of a VW bus. It wasn't your normal sexual lifestyle. Before we left Israel I'd begun working on my Ph.D. at the University of Jerusalem. My thesis had three parts. The first part I completed in Italy, the second I did in southern France, and I planned on doing the final third in California. They're all Mediterranean climates. I specialized in certain types of vegetation that thrived in Mediterranean environments. We were traveling around and I had to cobble my thesis into shape.

When we came to the United States, we drove across the country. We lived in California and I worked for nearly eighteen months in San Diego. We worried constantly about money. I was an errant scholar, always struggling to finish my dissertation, and we fretted about our immigration status. There was always stress. We really didn't know what normal life was like.

THERE'S SOMETHING WRONG HERE

Things changed in 1985 when I finally got my Ph.D. This was going to be the beginning of a normal life for us. I got a good postdoctoral position at MIT, which lasted for a year, and then found another position at Boston University. Our immigration status wasn't so up in the air, we began earning enough money to eliminate those worries, our work eased off—we started to have a normal life. And yet there were still the sexual hassles. So we said, OK, all those things are out of the way, there's something wrong here.

During this entire period of eight or ten years, it required more and more relaxation for me to be able to have satisfactory sex, to have an orgasm. Becky was an absolute gem about it. She has what seem to me very easy and very sound sexual responses. She's always been able to have orgasms. We always found that emotional closeness, obviously, was critical.

My physical difficulty was that my penis was often just not hard enough to be stimulated by her vagina. Vaginal manipulation had to be very intense for me to have an orgasm, and I had to have not had an orgasm for a week or two beforehand. When I look back on it, it was a gradual decline. Every time we would get relaxed and everything would seem fine, it was more and more difficult for me to have a proper erection.

We had never really considered trying to get medical help, because all the stuff we'd heard was that impotence is 90 percent in your head. We both didn't know enough. In 1987, I finally decided there's definitely something going on here.

I went to see my doctor and I told him. I went to him for something else—I'd injured my shoulder and I just wanted some advice about it. Then I mentioned in passing that I thought I might have a problem with impotence, something physically wrong with my erections. Intense feelings in the tip of my penis would last only briefly, and then my erection would diminish.

My doctor said, "No, no. You know the vagina is very lubricated. Of course the feeling in your penis goes down as the friction decreases, so if your penis was hard to begin with, and you were aroused, your erection might soften." He added, "That happens to me, too."

He went on to cite the same figures that my wife and I had heard, that something like 90 percent of impotence has to do with psychological factors. I went home and I told Becky, "Well, he just thinks it's a psychological problem of some sort." So, we left it at that.

This was in January of 1987. In July, I returned to the same practice for further treatment for my shoulder. The doctor I had seen previously had left the practice. I saw his partner, an Israeli, a fellow countryman, same medical school as the university where I was trained. I liked him straight off. He wanted to give me a general medical exam, since I'd never had one. I went back a few weeks later for my shoulder exercises and I mentioned to him that I still had this problem and recounted the response of his former partner.

This doctor was wonderful. He said, "Well, you may have a problem, but let's approach this in the correct way. There's a lot that can be done now. We'll tackle this as a medical thing first. If there is a medical problem, we'll clear that out of the way, and then figure out what to do for the psychological end of the story." He immediately drew some blood to do hormone levels, prolactin, testosterone, all that stuff, and then he sent me to Dr. Goldstein's practice, where I was ultimately treated. That was about October or November of 1987.

LOOKING BACK:
A PSYCHOLOGICAL CAUSE?

Aside from the obvious benefits to our lovemaking, what most interests me about tackling my impotence problem was how it jarred loose little pieces of my past, partially occluded memories.

Given my background, my home life, I had good reason for thinking there might be a psychological cause for my impotence.

Both my parents were immigrants to Israel. My mother was Hungarian; my father, Greek. My father was abusive and violent toward my mother, with the whole macho Mediterranean mindset in his attitudes toward women. He had an awful view of women.

Once they were having a fight in their bedroom, which was right next to ours, and there was all this yelling. The door was shut, but my brother and I could hear them screaming at each other. There was the sound of thumping, followed by silence, then a horrible noise. My brother and I—we must have only been eight and nine, since it was before their divorce—roared into their room. My father was sitting on top of my mother, with the telephone cord around her neck, strangling her.

We kicked him. I remember screaming and kicking him in the face and that must have been enough to rouse him. I don't think he actually knew what he was doing.

My brother and I—my brother's only fifteen months younger than I am—used to play in a sandbox together, and we used to play with our penises (not with each other's, but just each playing with his own penis), and we used to get erections. But, when his penis used to get an erection, he used to get up and get out of the box when he was done and he'd still have an erection. I noticed that mine used to go up and then go down. I was afraid that there was something different about my penis.

I didn't discuss any of this with my parents. I didn't dare go near my father with sexual problems. My mother tended to be relaxed about that subject, but I also knew she was hugely concerned about our health—if there had been anything wrong, she would have been all in a frenzy about it.

To compound things, I was sexually abused when I was fourteen by a man in a clothing store. We wore uniforms at my school, and

I was sent to get my uniform for the current year. This man–he was only about twenty or twenty-one–sexually abused me in the changing room and I didn't know what to do.

It was an overwhelmingly weird experience for me, accompanied by feelings of shame and self-hate, and of not understanding why I'd been singled out. Also, not being quite sure of what was going on with my penis, I thought maybe the reason that this happened was because I really was gay.

That possibility drifted all the way through my history. I used to think, "Maybe my penis doesn't really work well because I had sex with a man. Maybe if I become homosexual, that will solve the problem." I experimented with gay sex during adolescence and just afterward, in my very early twenties. I really didn't like it. I liked the closeness with the men–that was a big contradiction for me compared to the lack of closeness that I had with my father.

I know now that I was trying to figure out if my penis would function better in a gay situation. It didn't make any difference, but then I didn't know if that was because I was feeling bad about homosexuality or because I had some other problem.

In any event, by adolescence, I had this huge fear of relationships. I did have girlfriends, but because of my worry about my penis, I made sure that I had girlfriends with whom my chances of having a sexual encounter were small. That was a conscious decision. I remember laughing at myself, almost sardonically, thinking in my head, "I know why you're trying to avoid this."

I remember one high school girl, Shoshona. She was the first girl that I met in high school and we actually ended up being in college together, too. We both got interested in the same things, and I remained friends with her on and off.

She had other boyfriends, but I'm sure she wasn't sexual with them either. At some level she had made a decision to preserve her virginity for marriage. I must have sensed this–kids are really smart about this stuff. I must have known that she was like this, that having sex with her was unlikely.

At university I had another girlfriend whose name was Michelle, and she was both old-fashioned and worldly at the same time. I suspect that she had the same views as Shoshona, although we didn't really talk about sex. She died at a certain point in our relationship–she was murdered in her apartment. It was awful. She died just before I met Becky.

In 1980 I got involved in "co-counseling," a program in which peers provide nonprofessional counseling for each other. It started in San Diego and it's pretty much worldwide now. The participants come from every possible class and intellectual background.

The theory holds that you know and understand everything about yourself, but you just need someone to listen and encourage you to talk and figure things out. The co-counseling program stressed that human beings tend to behave in accordance with certain principles, and that most problems in behavior occur as a result of having been hurt.

I was often confused about myself, about how my family had affected me, why I was impotent, but at least I had this counseling to fall back on, to help me deal with my emotional issues.

During the first period of my relationship with Becky, I had all the traditional worries and fears associated with impotence, feeling less a man, plunging into depression because of society's odd notions of masculinity, which I completely bought at the time. Here was somebody whom I really loved, to whom I was sexually attracted—bar none—yet I couldn't sustain an erection with her. I just didn't understand it and I thought there must be something wrong with me.

Yet my relationship with Becky had too much going for it for me to want to leave it. It would have been an absolutely dreadful waste to have even considered leaving it.

I decided—and the co-counseling helped a lot—that, first of all, life is much bigger than just sex. We spend so much time just thinking about the distinctions, about being gay or being straight or bisexual or whatever. We characterize our lifestyles by an activity that probably occupies about five minutes a day. It's irrational.

You know, we don't say, "I'm a botanist and it's a lifestyle," although I certainly spend fourteen hours a day thinking about botany in one form or another. It seemed bizarre to me that we should emphasize sex so much, so I was able rationally and also emotionally to put it aside.

LOOKING BACK: A PHYSICAL CAUSE?

In disentangling my sexual confusion, I eventually came to believe that there was probably a physical component to all of my sexual troubles. By 1987, I'd been digging around for six or seven years, long enough that I felt pretty good about myself, and the more I continued digging the more certain I felt that there wasn't any giant catharsis waiting for me to discover.

After a while you trust yourself; you say, if this is capable of being figured out then I would have figured it out by now. I have enough belief in my own soundness to say that the physical problem was the only thing it could be.

In addition to all the psychological stuff, I also remembered physical injuries to my crotch when I was young, and I began to think they might have impaired my functioning.

I don't know if I was six or seven or eight, somewhere in that period, when my brother and a friend of his and I were fooling around on the trunk of an old-fashioned car. In those days the keyhole protruded quite far; it was a chrome-covered thing. We were sliding off the rear windshield and down the trunk and I misjudged the angle. I slipped backwards and I actually remember hooking my crotch against this keyhole. I fell off over the fender and onto the ground.

We all laughed, but I remember thinking that I'd actually ripped my crotch. I stuck my hand into my pants, fully expecting to feel blood because I had this warm, burning sensation all around the inside of my crotch. There was nothing there, but I was in pain. The pain didn't just subside, like when you hit yourself hard and then the pain fades. The rest of the time we were playing I kept rubbing my legs together my crotch hurt so much.

Later, when I was at school, I did some gymnastics and the first time I tried parallel bars, I didn't have enough strength in my arms and I fell sideways onto the same area of my crotch where I had previously been injured with the keyhole.

I finally decided, "OK, I'll tell this to my general practitioner, to my own doctor, and see what comes of it."

DIAGNOSIS

My family doctor believed that the first step toward curing my impotence was a physical workup. He wasn't an expert on impotence, but he did some basic blood tests and then sent me to Dr. Goldstein's practice. That was about October or November of 1987.

My hormone levels, which my doctor had tested, were fine. They ran some additional tests at Dr. Goldstein's clinic, ruling out neurological problems, and then scheduled me for a DICC study [DICC studies are sophisticated tests of the erectile mechanisms described in detail in the box on page 102.] To run this study, they inject your penis with papaverine and phentolamine, drugs that induce an erection. [Phentolamine blocks the constriction of the smooth muscles of the erection chambers.] Then they pump a saline solution (sounds horrible, but it's painless) into your penis.

The people who performed the study were not quite able to disguise their amazement at how much venous [from veins] leakage there was in my penis. Dr. Goldstein later told me it was probably due to the damage done by old injuries to my crotch. They couldn't pump the saline fast enough to even get my penis fully erect. They located most of the problem in the hidden part of my penis, under my crotch—that's where the veins were the most open when they were supposed to be squeezed shut by underlying, expanded erectile tissue.

I was amazed, and overwhelmed with relief at having a physical problem so dramatically confirmed. Becky picked me up in our car. I was so overwrought I burst into tears and cried all the way back to work. Becky didn't show very much emotion at the time. Since then she's apologized for misunderstanding me, for thinking that it was all psychological. In a way, she misjudged me slightly—both of us did. Anyway, she was relieved when we got the test results.

A short time later an arteriogram [see box, page 78] was performed, and they found extensive blockage in several important penile arteries, also located in the hidden part of my penis. In short, my penis was slow to fill with blood, because of the arterial blockage; and when the blood did finally fill my penis, I had trouble storing it.

I went to discuss the results of the test data with Dr. Goldstein a week after my arteriogram. "Did you ever hurt yourself—do you remember ever falling?" he asked.

I told him about falling from the car trunk as a young child; later came the fall from a set of parallel bars; in between I had tumbled off the roof of our house into the flower bed. There were several other incidents that probably also contributed to what happened there.

TREATMENT

The suggested treatment was a two-in-one surgery: to tie off all the places where my veins were draining to control the storage problem, and then to take an unblocked artery out of my abdominal wall and connect it to the penile artery to increase the amount of blood flow to my penis. Given the evidence of my tests, this seemed perfectly logical to Becky and me. I was given a date for surgery in early April.

Becky took me to the hospital on the morning of April 4, 1988. She accompanied me as far the antiseptic area, then wished me luck. Dr. Goldstein's team was very receptive to my aversion to general anesthesia. I wanted the absolute minimum amount of drugs, and nobody argued with me. Personally, I think that anesthetic drugs interfere with subsequent healing and subsequent function. I would rather endure the pain, as well as deal with it emotionally, at the time of the event.

My attitude was also connected to the fact that I'm a scientist by training and I'm interested in the process. I wanted to know exactly what they were doing and why they were doing it. So, while I certainly wanted anesthesia, I didn't want to be completely under. Dr. Goldstein was quite wonderful in that respect, without being paternalistic or evasive.

I went into the operating room and I was there from 7:15 in the morning till about 4:00 the afternoon, on my back the entire time. I had an epidural anesthetic. [*Epidural* anesthesia deadens the nerves coming from the lower spinal cord without causing the patient to lose consciousness.] They replenished the anesthetic twice. We had a great day. We spent quite a lot of the morning listening to the radio and then talking about science.

I really wanted to see what they were doing. They didn't have a mirror, but at one point Dr. Goldstein had his assistants prop my head up so I could looking over the surgical screen. I could actually see what they were doing to my penis — it was fascinating.

They devoted the morning session, until about 12:30, to tying off the abnormally draining veins so that I could store blood more effectively in my penis during an erection. In the afternoon, they opened my abdominal wall, severed the end of an artery, transferred the end into my groin and connected it to the arteries in my penis. The end of the artery split into two blood vessels. They connected one to each of the penile arteries, because both of mine were partly occluded. This part of the procedure was to increase blood flow to the penis — to correct what Dr. Goldstein calls "failure to fill."

At Dr. Goldstein's suggestion I dozed off for a while; my movements while awake were making it difficult to stitch the microscopic sutures for the arterial connections.

Three days after the surgery I started having morning erections. It had been so long since that happened I couldn't remember when I'd previously had one. Becky and I were forbidden to have sex for six weeks. The new connections to the penile arteries needed to heal; premature intercourse could have damaged them.

After two weeks I was getting very hard erections. They woke me up at night because they were actually painful. Tissue was probably being stretched in ways it hadn't been stretched before, because now it was able to store the blood more effectively. After about three weeks my penis felt great, and then after six weeks we could have sex. It was a whole lot better, unbelievably different.

But it was already clear that my erections at six weeks were not what they had been at three. My erections continued to decline, so Dr. Goldstein put me on a self-injection program, using papaverine and phentolamine.

I started off with small doses. The dose worked fine two or three times, but then was inadequate. I tried higher and higher doses, until eventually I was injecting over twice my original dosage. When that didn't do the trick we shifted course slightly, using prostaglandin E1, a new drug first introduced in Japan and Europe. [*Prostaglandin E1* relaxes the smooth-muscle tissue in the erection chambers.]

I was one of the first patients in Dr. Goldstein's clinic to be given prostaglandin El.

For the first few minutes following the injection, nothing happened. Then I could feel my penis starting to expand. I was at the clinic so they could see what happened. Fifteen minutes of excruciating pain followed, with some bleeding. On the elevator down to the street the pain became so bad I almost fainted, but as soon as I sat down the pain subsided. Anyway, the long and the short of it was that prostaglandin El didn't work for me either.

A SECOND OPERATION

After a second DICC study, they found that I still had leakage, around the lowest part of my penis. I was leaking from the big veins that arise from the hidden part of the penis. [This hidden part of the penis is called the *crus* (see illustration, page 11)]. Three or four of them could be seen in an X ray; they were each as big as my pinkie finger. The blood that was supposed to be holding up my erections was leaking out through my veins on its way back to my heart.

Dr. Goldstein suggested trying a new procedure that he had been researching. He had a hunch that the problem with me was partly in my erectile tissue itself—that it had been damaged in my various accidents and therefore couldn't expand to compress my penile veins. He suggested that this new procedure, called a "crural plication" or "crural tuck," would tighten the covering around the corpora cavernosa and enable compression of the veins without the erectile tissue inside having to expand very much.

I agreed to try a second operation, and we scheduled it for several months later.

———— ◆ ————

The second surgery was very brief. I went into the hospital in the morning, the procedure took less than an hour, and I went home that evening.

I woke up at about one a.m. with an extremely painful erection. I took a nonprescription pain medication to go to sleep, but nothing else. The night erections were painful at first, but that wore off. I didn't have a strong morning erection without pain till about two months after. Becky and I didn't have sex for a month—doctor's orders. Dr. Goldstein wanted to make sure that the healing was absolutely optimal.

The operation made a huge difference. I still have both morning and night erections. My erections aren't perfect, but they're much, much improved. When erect, my penis points straight out (if I'm standing), rather than straight up. But the main thing is that the head of my penis stays completely hard now, so that my sensations are much more stimulating, much more intense, and they lead to orgasm. As far as I'm concerned, my sexual functioning is 80 or 90 percent of what it should be. Both Becky and I are very happy. In fact, we are fortunate have our first child.

START WITH THE PHYSICAL

It's ironic, but I'm very glad that I didn't try to get assistance sooner somewhere else. This whole field is so new, had I tried to get help, say, ten years ago, I might have ended up spending money on people who were incapable of helping me.

In many ways, I'm very glad I hung out this long and didn't try to get any help from traditional psychotherapists—what would they have done? I would have gone over my whole history again and again and again. That might have helped me psychologically, but not done anything for my impotence. It could have been very discouraging.

The only advice I can offer someone with the same problem is to begin with a physical examination. Begin with the assumption your problem's physical. Even if you're absolutely sure that it's psychological, drop the assumption long enough to go and get all the necessary tests. The conventional wisdom holds that most of impotence is psychological, but that's simply not true.

Dr. Irwin Goldstein: The Medical Perspective

David, the man in this story, came to me as a thirty-eight-year-old Israeli immigrant with a long history of erection problems. His treatment reflects the rapid advances made in the surgical response to impotence in just the last few years.

Over the two-year period of David's treatment we gained some startling insights into the vascular mechanisms of erections. We also learned how to translate those insights into surgical techniques that restored his potency. As urology continues to expand its knowledge of erectile physiology, even greater numbers of impotent men will be able to avail themselves of increasingly effective surgical techniques.

David first sought medical help for his impotence in 1987, when he was referred to me by his family doctor. During his first visit I learned that he had undergone extensive counseling, both alone and with his wife, with no discernable improvement in his potency.

David's medical history didn't include high cholesterol, high blood pressure, cigarette smoking, diabetes mellitus or any of the other vascular risk factors that might have interfered with his erectile physiology. Tests also failed to uncover anything unusual in his hormone levels or in the functioning of his nerves.

Based on his history and his tests, and the long duration of his problem, I suspected that we were dealing with the effects of some long-ago injury to his perineum, the area covering the hidden part of his penis. As David himself says in his narrative, once he began asking himself whether he had ever hurt that part of his body, memories of old accidents began coming back. For many men, a specific traumatic episode remains beyond conscious recall at first, either because it occurred so long ago, or because it appeared innocuous at the time it happened. David, who had only recently begun to consider the possible connection between injury and impotence, was able to recount in vivid detail several accidents from the first fifteen years of his life that I thought might account for his present problems.

BLOCKAGE AND LEAKAGE

I next ran a DICC study on David (see box, page 102).

The overwhelming majority of patients with organic impotence have problems with blood flow both into and out of the penis—in short, not enough blood comes into and too much blood leaves the penis during erection.

The blood-pressure levels in David's erectile chambers were just barely within the lowest limits of normal. David's tests revealed that one of the two main arteries that fed blood to his penis was closed off, while the other was about 50 percent blocked. The blockages were localized in the perineum (the area between the penis and the anus); the other arteries—outside the perineum—were normal. These blockages interfered with the supply of blood flowing to his penis.

As I discussed in chapter 2, a localized blockage is often the end product of an accidental injury that damages the lining of the artery. Blockages, similar to those in atheroclerosis, form at the site of the injury, obstructing the artery. Most likely David's fall while playing atop an automobile trunk as a small boy, as well as his other injuries, set up his particular blockages.

David's tests also uncovered abnormally high drainage of blood from the perineal section of his penis during erections. What blood was reaching his penis during arousal was rapidly flowing out of it.

The DICC Study

DICC, short for "dynamic infusion cavernosometry and cavernosography," is a four-part examination of a patient's erectile system during a drug-induced erection. It is a major tool in diagnosing the cause of impotence.

A DICC study begins with a physician injecting a large dose of both *papaverine* and *phentolamine* into the corpora cavernosa of the patient's penis. *Papaverine* is a chemical that relaxes the smooth-muscle tissue in the erectile chambers and penile arteries. *Phentolamine* blocks the constriction of smooth-muscle tissue and arteries that can be caused by the patient's own hormone *adrenaline* and the neurotransmitter *noradrenaline*. Adrenaline-like chemicals, such as adrenaline and noradrenaline, are released in large amounts when a patient is anxious.

The first part of the DICC study records the blood-pressure response in the corpora cavernosa of the patient's penis following the injection of papaverine and phentolamine. The physician is identifying how closely the penile blood pressure approaches the average or mean blood pressure of an artery in the patient's arm (see page 26).

The patient's storage mechanism is tested during the next phase of cavernosometry by infusing saline (salt) solution into the corpora cavernosa (erection chambers)— it's painless—until the patient's penis reaches a defined pressure in the erection chambers. The physician then charts how fast the erection pressure declines after the saline infusion is stopped. The normal, undamaged storage mechanism is quite efficient, and the flow of saline needed to maintain pressure and the erection pressure drop are both very small. If the patient's storage mechanism is not functioning, there will be a high flow of saline needed to maintain pressure in the erection chambers or a marked drop in penile pressure when the saline infusion is stopped.

In the third part of a DICC study, ultrasound is used to measure the blood pressure of the penile arteries, to see if pressure is adequate.

Cavernosography, the fourth and final part of the procedure, produces an X ray of the erect penis, providing the physician with vital anatomical information regarding the storage mechanism.

TREATMENT OPTIONS

What was to be done? There were four options for David's physiologic problems: a penile implant, penile injections, a vacuum constriction device or surgery. He had already had some counseling for the psychological aspects of his sexual problems, and we felt there was no need for further psychotherapy or sex therapy.

After brief discussion, David, Becky and I dismissed any thought of giving David an implant. The single most serious drawback to implants is their irreversibility. Implantation of a penile prosthesis destroys erectile tissue, forever eliminating any future possibility of restoring the patient's own erectile physiology.

In a middle-aged or older patient, or a man whose physiology will always be compromised by a disease (like diabetes mellitus, for example), an implant is a rational choice (I'll talk more about implants in chapter 7).

But for a young man in good health, I usually advise against an implant as a first line of treatment. I counsel patients to try other therapies first, to see if they can live with a less drastic alternative. Certainly the explosion of effective surgical treatments for impotence, undreamed of five years ago, makes waiting a rational choice. If there isn't a surgical cure for your impotence now, wait a little; there may be one shortly.

Injection treatments were another alternative. I explained the program to David and Becky, and, as you know from David's narrative, the injections were used only after surgery and did help him to some extent for a period of time. The prostaglandin E1 injection was not helpful in David's case. He did not like the vacuum constriction device.

The fourth option was surgery. David was quite fortunate in having localized arterial blockages. From the standpoint of a surgeon, whether blockages are localized or diffuse appears from our experience to be critical. In the procedure known as revascularization (see Tom's story in chapter 4), a surgeon can make small changes in the routes of a patient's arteries, bypassing localized blockage(s) and restoring a healthy flow of blood to the penis. When the blockages are diffuse, this usually isn't possible. David was an ideal candidate for revascularization. We could reroute his arterial blood flow around the scarred areas.

But, stopping his abnormal drainage would prove to be a bit trickier.

SURGERY

David and his wife opted for surgery.

As David described, we improved blood flow to his penis by

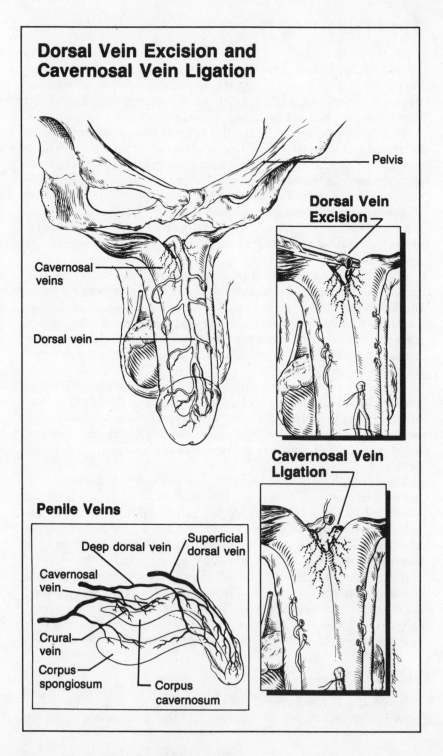

Dorsal Vein Excision and Cavernosal Vein Ligation

Pelvis

Dorsal Vein Excision

Cavernosal veins

Dorsal vein

Cavernosal Vein Ligation

Penile Veins

Deep dorsal vein

Superficial dorsal vein

Cavernosal vein

Crural vein

Corpus spongiosum

Corpus cavernosum

revascularization, rerouting an artery from his abdominal wall. This procedure was performed to correct David's filling problem.

At first, we thought we could solve David's storage problem by using *ligation;* that is, tying off some of the veins in his penis and excising (removing) the dorsal vein (see illustration, page 104). We did this during his first operation. Unfortunately, ligation of these veins was not sufficient to restore David's storage mechanism. Even with the extra blood flow from the revascularization, his penis still couldn't store enough blood for a dependable erection.

It just so happened that at the time I was treating David, the sixth annual meeting of the International Society for Impotence Research was taking place in Boston. At the meeting, Japanese scientists showed photographs, taken with a scanning electron microscope, of the tiny veins that drain the erectile tissues. I could, for the first time, actually see these structures coming off the outer edge of the erectile tissue. Seeing these structures for the first time in humans made it more obvious to me that, in a healthy man, the erectile tissue expands during arousal, mechanically closing these venules in the subtunical space against the tunica (see chapter 2, page 18 and illustration, page 21).

At the same meeting, other Japanese scientists demonstrated that aging was associated with the stiffening of erectile tissue. As erectile tissue becomes stiffer, less elastic, it becomes less able to expand to compress the venules against the tunica. The venules therefore remain open and "leak" blood out of an erection. The Japanese demonstrated that *collagen,* a fibrous protein material, could become deposited in erectile tissue and cause the tissue to become stiff and to lose its stretchiness. Collagen deposits are associated with aging, diabetes and vascular risk factors such as high cholesterol, but they are also associated with *scarring*—the kind of scarring caused by injuries like David's.

In David's case, I postulated that his childhood injury to his perineum had damaged not only his arteries in the perineal area, but also the erectile tissue itself at the rearmost portion of his corpora

---

"Failure-to-store" impotence can sometimes be treated with vascular reconstructive surgery in which the major veins draining the hidden portions of the penis, the cavernosal veins, are tied off (ligated). The cavernosal veins exit from each erection chamber in the region of the juncture of the two erection chambers. Above the cavernosal vein lies the dorsal vein, which is removed (excised). The remaining network of veins draining the penis is left intact. Such surgery is designed to decrease blood drainage from this portion of the penis and improves blood storage during erection. This operation is usually performed in conjunction with the tucking (plication) of the hidden portions of the penis (see illustration, page 107).

cavernosa. His scarred erectile tissue simply wasn't expanding sufficiently to fill the subtunical space.With this critical step in his storing mechanism disabled, his subtunical venules couldn't close. This accounted for the open veins we saw on his cavernosogram (see illustration, page 30).

At this time (the late 1980s), I had been researching different approaches to tightening the tunica albuginea (the white coat that surrounds the corpora cavernosa, described in chapter 2). Tightening the tunica makes the space under it–the "subtunical" space–smaller; the veins are therefore easier to compress.

I reasoned that if we tightened David's tunica, we could restore the storing mechanism that his accidents had crippled. His corpora cavernosa would only have to enlarge slightly for the mechanism to work.

A HAPPY ENDING

David's story has a happy ending. His second operation, a "tuck," as the operation has come to be called (in medical terms, it's known as a *crural plication*), was successful (see illustration, page 107). He didn't even have to spend the night in the hospital. He was able to achieve and sustain rigid erections soon after the surgery and over a year after surgery, they remain strong but require the concomitant use of penile injections to maintain the needed rigidity.

Dr. Alma Dell Smith– The Psychological Perspective

I am commenting on David Herzog's case, with his permission, on the basis of taped interviews, case notes and conversations with Dr. Goldstein.

David, like most impotent men, needed to arrive at an explanation for his problem, a way of understanding what was happening to him.

An unusually sensitive and reflective man, he looked back into his past for the seeds of his present problem. His father was clearly an abusive parent. Children raised in an abusive situation receive mixed signals. On the one hand, his father was the most convenient role model for male sexuality; on the other, his father was aggressive, dominating, often brutal and contemptuous of David's mother.

Many boys have homosexual experiences, with no harm done to their adult sexuality. But in David's case, his abusive father must have raised doubts in David's mind about what it meant to be a man. David was all too willing to assign the blame to himself when something

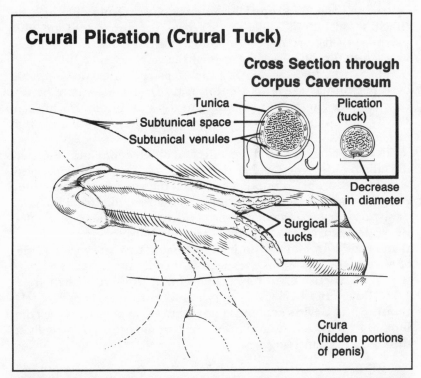

Crural Plication (Crural Tuck)

Cross Section through Corpus Cavernosum

Tunica
Subtunical space
Subtunical venules

Plication (tuck)

Decrease in diameter

Surgical tucks

Crura (hidden portions of penis)

"Failure-to-store" impotence may be treated by vascular reconstructive surgery in which the tunica around the crura (hidden portions of the penis) is plicated, or tucked. Such surgery helps close the subtunical space in this portion of the penis, thus decreasing leakage from the crural veins during erection. This operation is usually performed in conjunction with the tying off of the major veins draining the hidden portion of the penis (see illustration, page 104). It is indicated in cases where the erectile tissue cannot expand enough to fill the subtunical space and compress the subtunical venules.

went wrong—when his parents fought, when he was molested as an adolescent, when he was impotent with his future wife. Later, after he became involved in co-counseling, he began to see his way through some of the confusion about his background and identity.

When David met his wife, he was avoiding sexual feelings because he had lost a friend and had some unresolved feelings over early homosexual encounters. He believed his erectile difficulties were in part the consequence of his sexual experimentation. As David points out in his story, the commonly accepted wisdom was that most impotence was psychological in origin—and they accepted the common wisdom.

David and Becky never thought to question whether David might fit into that group of men with organic impotence. For seven years they blamed his problem on stress cause by external events—leaving

Israel, traveling to Europe and America, the pressure of exams and finishing his thesis — and David's own background of possible psychogenic factors. At that time, not once did it occur to them that an examination by a urologist might have been in order.

Yet, in order to overcome obstacles to psychological development, each person has to get to a point in his or her life where he can hear and see alternative explanations to assumptions. David's sensitivity and openness to reviewing painful experiences allowed him to consider co-counseling.

His counseling had no direct effect on his erections and ultimately led him to the conviction that something physical, not psychological, was at the heart of his impotence. But, at the same time, the counseling gave him a breadth of vision that preserved him from the utter devastation that so frequently visits the lives of impotent men. He and Becky decided, quite wisely, that their relationship was much larger than David's problems with his erections. Their story exemplifies how some couples, despite sexual dysfunction, nevertheless manage to sustain a sense of intimacy and mutual support in their lives.

For David and Becky, this story has a positive ending. The relationship and David's erections remain strong as a result of the combination of David's surgeries and the insights this couple gained through his counseling sessions.

CHAPTER 6

Norm —
The Injection Alternative

Norm Perkins (not his real name) first came to our clinic in 1987. At the time, he was in his early forties, married and a foreman in a truck factory. He successfully treats his impotence by giving himself injections that help induce an erection. As you will see, far from being unpleasant, penile injections are a safe, convenient, effective treatment.

Norm's Story

In 1980 I was mugged—I was beaten up, knocked to the ground and kicked several times in the crotch. Shortly after, I began losing my erections—they'd only last two or three minutes. I'd never had any problems before, but I never made any connection between being mugged and becoming impotent. At the time, my wife was having her own reproductive problems that made it difficult for her to become pregnant. I assumed my erection problems were somehow connected with my response to that. In subsequent years I blamed alcoholism; still later, I made an injury to my back the scapegoat for my erection difficulties.

My wife Gloria and I had been together for a long time—twenty-five years—when this happened. She and I started dating in high school. We went together for eight years before we were married. Not only did we have great sex, but we were best friends. Then suddenly, whammo—things didn't work.

We didn't really know what to do. We talked about my impotence. We cried about it. Impotence was something we were going to handle ourselves. We were a team, partners. You only get married once, no matter what problems come up—that was our attitude.

So, for seven years, twice a week, we tried to have intercourse. I'd get home and she'd meet me with nothing on, or a negligee. We'd try to make love and nothing would happen. She'd cry, convinced it was her fault. I'd say "It's not your fault—it's mine." We argued a lot. I knew something was wrong with me, but I didn't know what. It was a humiliating thing to deal with. We'd try and try, but I just couldn't get erect. It was tough watching her cry. I'd end up apologizing. The embarrassment was partially responsible for my delay in getting help. Our marriage got pretty bad, but we stuck it out.

DEPRESSION AND ALCOHOL

I spent a lot of those seven years depressed. Impotence made me feel like less of a man and I took to drinking to get rid of those feelings. A few years ago, I realized that alcohol wasn't a solution. I went through a private detox center, then entered counseling. I thought maybe my problem had something to do with my drinking, even though the problem had started before I began drinking—that's the kind of logic I was using. I also thought stress connected with our different schedules might might be contributing to the problem. I worked nights as a foreman for a truck company; Gloria had a day job. Maybe we just weren't connecting. Part of my difficulty was that nobody understood the problem, at least not anybody I ever ran into, including my counselor. Despite the counseling, I stayed impotent.

A TURNING POINT

Then, in 1986, I injured my back at the truck plant where I worked. We consulted an orthopedic surgeon, who operated on me later that year. He removed a couple of discs. At the time, I figured that the discs in my spine were compressing nerves to my penis—I assumed this, no one ever diagnosed it—and I hoped that after the surgery things would get better.

My sister came to visit me one day while I was recuperating. She's a hospital administrator. She had heard about Dr. Goldstein through the grapevine and she'd taken the trouble to call him up and explain my problem.

For some reason, for a brief time after I went home from the hospital, I was able to achieve a reasonable erection. Gloria and I even had intercourse. It was great. Unfortunately, the problem returned within a few weeks. We were crushed. But our disappointment had one good side effect—it wiped out my embarrassment about the problem. Something was wrong and I was determined to find out what it was. I got Dr. Goldstein's number from my sister and made an appointment.

A PHYSICAL PROBLEM

I have a vivid memory of my first visit to Dr. Goldstein's clinic. He put blood pressure cuffs on my arm and on my penis. He took both measurements and said, "This probably isn't psychological. There's really a strong chance you've got a physical problem. The blood pressure in your penile arteries is below normal."

A physical problem! Yahoo! It wasn't my fault! I can't tell you how good that made me feel. Things were looking up.

On my next visit I had more tests. They injected my penis with papaverine and phentolamine, which gave me a partial erection. Dr. Goldstein did a DICC study [see box, page 102] on me and rechecked the low blood flow during a similar drug-induced erection that was part of the study. Afterwards, he told me I also had an abnormality with the storage mechanism of my erection, especially in the hidden part of my penis. My last test was an arteriogram [see box, page 78] of my penis.

INJECTIONS

Dr. Goldstein and I talked about sex therapy and a vacuum device that can give you erections, but neither of those choices interested my wife and me. He also said an operation might be able to fix it, but Gloria was terrified of my having surgery. Dr. Goldstein then suggested I try papaverine and phentolamine injections. That sounded great to me.

The nurse gave me the penile shots the first five or six times. He started out with 0.15 milliliter (ml) of papaverine and phentolamine, then upped the dosage, first to 0.30 ml, and then to 0.60 ml. I think the maximum dosage in their office is 1.00 ml. I got up to 0.60 ml, which was close to the limit. They could only give me another 0.40 ml before I'd have to consider something else — maybe surgery.

Then he gave me 0.75 ml — the magic number. I was driving down the expressway on my way home when all of a sudden I started getting an erection.

I drove home at about a hundred miles an hour. Gloria was waiting for me, unsure if this time the shot was going to be successful or not. One look at my face told her that we'd hit the jackpot. We made love right away. I hadn't had a good erection in a couple of years, and that one lasted forty-five minutes. It was great! We were just was so happy! They increased my dosage to 0.80 ml, where it's stayed.

If a man with a healthy erection system took what I take, it would give him what Dr. Goldstein calls a "priapistic erection" — a prolonged erection. [*Priapism* is a condition of prolonged, painful erection that fails to subside (see pages 120 and 159).] You have to take what's good for you and they have to work you up real slowly.

The injection itself isn't bad—although injecting your penis has a few drawbacks. I got the hang of it pretty quickly. I learned how to locate an injection site at the side of the base of the penis. I clean the injection site with an alcohol swab, then fill an insulin syringe with 0.80 ml of the drug. I'm very careful to follow the exact dosage. I position the needle at a right angle to the sterilized skin covering my erection chamber. Then I insert the needle through the skin into the erection chamber and slowly inject the drug. After removing the needle I press the injection site for three to five minutes to prevent any bleeding. I cap the needle, dispose of it in a special plastic screw-top container I keep in the bathroom and return the bottle of papaverine and phentolamine to the refrigerator for cold storage. Ten minutes after the injection I'm a winner.

Most guys squirm when I first tell them about the shots, but the injections really don't hurt much. I tell them a story I once heard about an old lady who lived out in the woods. She had a still way down a hill in back of her house. She used to walk down the hill through three feet of snow every morning just to fill her little jug with white lightning. Somebody once said to her, "Doesn't it bother you, trudging through the snow every morning, just to get that bottle?" She said, "Yeah, but the way I feel on the way back makes up for the way I felt on the way down." That's how I feel about injecting myself. Cleaning your penis, injecting yourself and then compressing the injection site takes under ten minutes. The erection usually develops ten to fifteen minutes after the injection, especially with good foreplay. [Some patients find they need to wait as long as thirty minutes after an injection for a full erection to develop.] Gloria and I can both live with that.

Self-injection therapy turned my life around. After Dr. Goldstein treated me, I realized I should have thought about my erection problem the way you think about a broken arm—something's wrong, you get it fixed. He's advised me to stay on the injections until they get a little more experience with surgical treatment for filling and storing problems like mine. Mine are apparently a little more complicated than some. The field is changing quickly. If he calls one of these days and says, "Look, I've really perfected this operation," I'll have surgery. Until then, the injections are fine with me.

I don't know if I'd be comfortable with penile injections if I were single. I've tried to figure that out, how you'd go about it. Gloria comes over and sits in my lap and says, "I think it's time for a shot." We have no problem talking like that. A husband and wife can do that. But what do you do if you're in a bar or a nightclub and you pick somebody up? I don't know how a single guy would deal with it.

Gloria's only hang-up is that she doesn't like to watch me inject myself. She just doesn't like needles.

TALK ABOUT IT

I understand now that if you've got a problem, you have to spit it out. You have to sit down and deal with it. After Gloria had her third operation for infertility, I said, "Look, who the hell wants to bring a kid into this world today anyway? There's enough of them around. We'll take a couple that are already out there." We ended up adopting two beautiful children.

That's the way I feel about impotence now. If something's wrong with your eye, you talk about it. If something's wrong with your penis, you should talk about that. What's the big deal? I've come to realize that if you don't talk about it, you don't get it fixed. I met a cop right after I started taking the injections. He listened to my story and then he said, "Gee, that sounds just like me!" I gave him Dr. Goldstein's number. What did he have to lose?

Being open about something like impotence is new for me. I came from an alcoholic family. They didn't talk—they yelled. Both of my parents were drinkers. I grew up with abuse—verbal and physical abuse—my dad beating up my mother and us kids. I used to take the whippings for my younger brothers. I threw my father out when I was eighteen years old. He'd broken my mother's arm. I swore that would never happen in my family and it never has. If there's a problem, we don't yell, we don't scream—we talk. I spank my daughters— when it's supposed to happen—but not often. I deal with things, but I don't make a big issue out of them.

Gloria and I have a great relationship. We met at a high-school party in 1964. She just walked by me and I grabbed her by the arm. I never saw her before in my life. Then I started dancing with her and I took her home. We went out a couple times, and then we started going together. Then I went in the service—three years in the Marines. When I came back we got married. She was twenty-one; I was twenty-two. We've had bad times and good times, but we've always been the best of friends. She's always hung in there with me, through my erection problems, through the alcoholism. Even during the worst times, she was sympathetic because of her own problem with infertility. She doesn't blame herself anymore. The fact that I can't keep an erection without the drug doesn't upset her. I'm incredibly lucky to be married to her.

I love coming home each day. I can sit in my chair and my youngest daughter—she's eight—will go by me on her way upstairs. She'll turn around, come back and give me a hug, for no reason.

Since I went to Dr. Goldstein, I've stopped taking antacids and I no longer drink. I'm relaxed, back to a normal life, back to where I was when I got married.

Dr. Irwin Goldstein: The Medical Perspective

Norm Perkins first came to see me in February of 1987. He was a burly man in his early forties who calmly answered my questions about his background, marriage and sex life. By profession, he was a foreman in a truck factory outside of Boston. He had a hearty friendliness that I suspect made him a good manager.

I immediately liked Norm. He had a sense of practicality about him that I associate with people who've taken the time to consider what's really important in life. His wife Gloria had undergone several major surgical procedures in an unsuccessful attempt to restore her fertility. That had been followed by Norm's inability to maintain an erection, and later his battle with alcoholism. So many patients come to urologists in a state of desperation. "Make me potent," they cry, "or my marriage will fall apart!" Couples like Norm and Gloria, or David and Becky of chapter 5, who manage to remain intimate and committed to each other year after year despite the erection problems, are much more likely than less committed couples to have a successful outcome to their impotence treatment.

VASCULAR RISK FACTORS — AND AN INJURY

Norm had a long history of vascular risk factors. He was a heavy smoker with elevated cholesterol levels and he had pain in his legs when he exercised (often a sign of circulatory problems).

Researchers now theorize that an injured vascular system in the perineum is especially vulnerable to the effects of risk factors like smoking, elevated cholesterol levels and high blood pressure.

What concerned me most in Norm's case was a vicious mugging, during which he'd been brutally kicked several times in the perineum. It was extremely likely that this event had damaged the endothelial lining of the arteries in the hidden part of his penis. His lifestyle would only have made things worse. His smoking, high blood pressure and high cholesterol levels, according to present thinking, would have increased the likelihood of blood-vessel and erectile-tissue scarring at the places where he was kicked during the mugging.

A DICC study (see box, page 102) and an arteriogram (see box, page 78) confirmed Norm's vascular problems. He had blockages in the arteries that bring blood to the penis, and to some extent in the arteries within the erection chambers themselves. Also, as commonly happens in such cases, he had excessive drainage of blood away from his penis via open veins that should have been closed during an erection. In short, like many patients, Norm had problems with both his filling and his storage mechanisms.

NERVE PROBLEMS

Nerve problems further complicated his erectile physiology. Two types of nerves are involved in the erection process: *peripheral sensory* nerves, which register touch in the skin of the penis, particularly the *glans*, the sensitive head of the penis; and *motor autonomic* nerves, which tell the smooth-muscle tissue of the lacunar spaces to relax, thereby allowing the penis to fill with blood and bring the storing mechanism into play (see illustration, page 13).

Norm complained of numbness in the tip of his penis, an indicator of sensory-nerve damage, a frequent side effect of alcohol abuse. In addition, Norm had spinal disc problems. Further neurophysiologic testing with a neurologist confirmed that Norm did indeed have some minor sensory-nerve impairment in his glans. The real question was whether there was damage to the motor autonomic nerves in addition to sensory-nerve damage. There was a real chance that either neurologic problem—damage from alcoholism or his disc problem—might also have affected his important motor autonomic nerves.

TREATMENT OPTIONS

Norm readily agreed to quit smoking and go on a diet in order to lose weight and reduce his cholesterol levels. While I knew these lifestyle changes would help lessen the likelihood of further damage to his erectile physiology, they wouldn't repair the vascular damage that had already been done. Surgery might help. Given the evidence of his DICC study and arteriogram, he looked like a reasonable candidate for vascular reconstructive surgery. I felt confident we could bypass the majority of his arterial blockages, but we were less confident we could improve his storage mechanism. And, this would still leave the real problem of his impaired sensory nerves, and the potential problem of his untestable motor autonomic nerves.

This left four alternatives—sex therapy, the vacuum constriction device, an implant or penile injections. Norm and Gloria rejected sex therapy, and neither of them liked the vacuum device. Too much of Norm's own erectile functioning seemed intact for me to recommend an implant.

Penile injections are a predictable, rational, successful and safe treatment; usually there are minimal side effects. Unlike a younger couple, who might have felt a greater necessity to repair surgically the man's own functioning, Norm and Gloria were willing to try incorporating injection therapy into their love life. They recognized that the most important issue for them was restoring their ability to have intercourse, with as little complication as possible. All things considered, penile injections made the most sense to them as a remedy for the present. They decided to consider surgery at a later date, if and when the outcome became more predictable for cases like Norm's. Norm enrolled in the clinic's injection program.

Norm's response to self-injections wasn't completely without anxiety—what man willingly wants to stick a needle, even a very small one, into his penis? But Norm soon adjusted. His wife smoothed the way by maintaining an open and encouraging attitude, and a sense of humor. Now, almost three and a half years later, both of them are still doing fine. For Norm and Gloria, the injections were a small price to pay for the return of their love life.

Self-Injection Therapy

by Terry Payton, R.N., B.S.

Terry Payton is a nurse clinician and clinical coordinator in the Department of Urology at University Hospital in Boston who helped develop and implement the self-injection program at the Center.

In 1983 North American urologists at a convention in Las Vegas received a starling demonstration of the efficacy of drug-induced erection. During an evening seminar, a British researcher rose to present a lecture on the physiology of erection. His audience was composed of several hundred urologists jammed into a large conference room. Unlike previous speakers at the meeting, the guest lecturer was dressed in a pair of loose-fitting sweatpants.

Approximately thirty minutes into his presentation, he remarked that, in fact, at that very moment, his own penis was getting hard. Most of the urologists chuckled, thinking he was joking. A few more minutes passed. Suddenly he stopped, then said, "I must demonstrate this." He stepped out from behind the lectern and lowered his sweatpants, revealing his own penis in a state of blazing rigidity. He then wandered among the first few rows of the audience, inviting the astonished urologists to palpate his erection. He wanted them to confirm for themselves that his penis was indeed quite rigid—without the use of an implant.

Despite the unorthodox presentation, the era of penile injections was ushered into being. His erection was induced by a drug injected into his penis, a drug similar to the ones used by impotent men today. Since then, drugs that induce erections have revolutionized impotence diagnosis with the advent of the DICC study. Self-injection therapy has also proven an effective, attractive treatment option for many men, such as Norm Perkins, either on a permanent basis or as an interim measure while a man considers surgery, or even to help improve erections after surgery.

The most commonly used drugs have been *papaverine* and *phentolamine.* Papaverine itself acts directly on the smooth-muscle tissue of the penis, relaxing the walls of the penile arteries and erectile lacunar spaces in order to increase blood flow into the penis (see illustration, page 13). The erectile tissue then expands against the tunica, enabling the penis to store blood (see illustration, page 21). The net result is an erection. Phentolamine, a drug that blocks the constricting action of the sympathetic nervous system on the erectile tissue, is often mixed with papaverine. This helps sustain the erection and make the papaverine more effective. Other drugs, such as *prostaglandin E1,* can be used alone or be added to papaverine and phentolamine to increase their effectiveness.

Prostaglandin E1, like papaverine, directly relaxes the smooth-muscle tissue of the penis. It has an advantage over papaverine and phentolamine in that it is metabolized (broken down) in the penis itself rather than in the liver. (Other drugs, such as papaverine, are broken down in the liver, where they rarely cause allergic or hypersensitive reactions.) Some men report pain or a burning sensation in the penis shortly after injection. Prostaglandin E1 is the latest addition to the list of drugs becoming available for penile injections and is the first to become FDA approved for the treatment of impotence. Probably, even more effective drugs to promote an erection will be discovered in the future. In other countries, combinations of multiple drugs are being developed, with results that surpass any of the single-drug or two-drug regimens now in common use in the United States.

A very small needle is used for a penile injection. The injection itself is relatively painless. For most patients the greatest discomfort is the psychological hurdle of learning to inject themselves in the penis. After injection, a patient's penis will usually start to become erect within ten to fifteen minutes. Almost all patients will develop an erection within thirty minutes. From the standpoint of appearance and sensation, there's little or no difference between an "ordinary" erection and one that results from an injection, although there may be less swelling of the glans in an injection-induced erection. The erection itself lasts between thirty minutes and an hour (a bonus-

many men find that ejaculation will not cause them to lose their erection). Patients are advised to use common sense concerning the frequency of use–never more than once in the same day. The average patient uses penile injections twice a week.

Patients learn how to administer the drug through a carefully supervised program involving training and follow-up visits to the clinic. Over the course of several visits the lowest volume of drug–or drug combinations–that will still initiate and maintain an erection is determined. The dosage is much lower than that administered for diagnostic reasons.

The patient then learns how to inject himself properly (in many cases, we've taught women how to inject their partners' penises). He learns how to prevent himself from injecting himself in the wrong places, like the urinary passageway or the nerves and blood vessels at the top of the penis (see illustration, page 119). He is also taught the importance of compressing the injection site for three to five minutes. Compression minimizes internal bleeding, theoretically diminishing any chance of scarring. All of this may sound daunting, but the overwhelming majority of men for whom the injections are effective soon master the process.

IS INJECTION THERAPY FOR EVERYONE?

A wide variety of patients responds well to injection therapy. The drugs used in penile injections mimic what happens during the initial stage of arousal; that is, they cause the smooth-muscle tissue of the penis to dilate. It follows that the patients who respond best to injection therapy are those who have trouble during the first stage of the erection process–"initiating." These patients frequently have nerve damage; their smooth-muscle tissue never gets the signal to relax. Penile injections with low dosages are often quite effective in restoring the potency of these men.

Injection therapy has also been useful in patients with vascular problems, including arterial blockages and abnormal storage capabilities. Sometimes penile injections can provide just enough of a boost to compensate for the damage–if it's not too severe–to the patient's filling and storing mechanisms.

Finally, injection therapy may be a useful alternative for patients with psychogenic impotence when sex therapy is not helpful, or it may be used as a temporary adjunct to sex therapy.

In our experience, self-injections, like all treatments for impotence, work best when a man has a supportive partner. Embarrassment, psychological discomfort, the "artificiality" of the process – all of these can be overcome when both partners receive

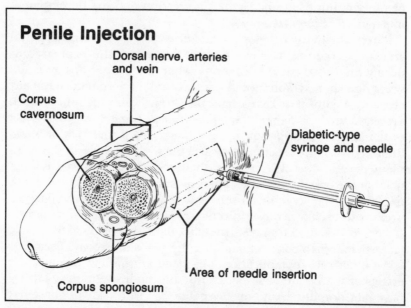

Penile Injection

Dorsal nerve, arteries
and vein

Corpus
cavernosum

Diabetic-type
syringe and needle

Area of needle insertion

Corpus spongiosum

Drugs that promote smooth-muscle relaxation and erection can be injected into the erection chambers. The injection is performed with a needle of small
gauge, similar to the equipment used by patients injecting insulin for treatment
of diabetes.

full information concerning the proper administration and use of
the injections. Norm and Gloria, for example, with their affec-
tionately humorous "Time for a shot" demonstrate how injections
may be happily integrated into a couple's love life.

Some women have complained of feeling uninvolved when a husband disappears into the bathroom, emerging a few minutes later
with a full erection. They feel as though their desirability had little
or nothing to do with stimulating their husbands. Consequently, we
sometimes counsel men to wait until after a period of foreplay before
giving themselves an injection. Also, we sometimes like to adjust the
dosage so that it gives a man about 60 percent of his erection, relying on the stimulation of lovemaking to provide him with the rest.

Most of the potential problems with the injections are avoided
by the training process that patients go through when they become
part of the injection program. During the training period, patients
learn how to use the medications safely, how to inject themselves
properly, how to utilize the minimum dosage necessary to achieve
a satisfactory erection and how to recognize complications. However,
self-injection does present certain risks, including scarring of the

penis, bending of the penis during erection and the development of *priapistic erections* (see below).

Rarely, a man will develop a *priapistic erection,* a prolonged, painful erection, as the result of an injection. But usually this happens only during the initial period of therapy when the proper dosage is still being determined. You should notify your doctor immediately if any erection is painful or lasts longer than four hours (painful or not). *Prolonged erections can result in lasting damage to the erectile tissue if not treated in time.* With priapism, the danger lies in the lack of blood drainage from the erectile tissue and the high pressure in the erectile tissue shutting off the artery that feeds the tissue. Pain is a signal that the erectile tissue isn't getting enough arterial blood. If left untreated, the erectile tissue may be permanently damaged. Treatment usually involves injection of an adrenaline-like drug into the erectile tissue. This causes the smooth-muscle tissue of the penile lacunar spaces to contract, allowing the penis to become flaccid.

Another rare complication of injection therapy involves the effects of the penile drug papaverine on the liver. In our clinic we have monitored the patients' liver function with tests and have not experienced any problems.

The long-term effects of self-injection are unknown. The practice of self-injection hasn't been around long enough for scientists to gauge its effects fifteen or twenty years down the road. At present, there are approximately 100,000 American men using penile injections; on average, they use them twice a week. Since 1983, many millions of penile injections have been administered in the United States and around the world. To my knowledge, there has been only one reported death associated with an erection-inducing drug, blood clots formed during a prolonged erection were the apparent cause.

Most potential problems are avoided by the screening process that precedes acceptance into a program.

If you'd like to consider penile injections, you should consult with a urologist who specializes in impotence and who has had experience with self-injection therapy. Treated with respect, penile injections can safely and effectively restore a couple's love life with relatively little inconvenience or risk and can often substitute for vascular or implant surgery.

Dr. Alma Dell Smith— The Psychological Perspective

I evaluated Norm and Gloria Perkins to determine what, if any,

The FDA and
Penile Injectable Medications

All the drugs used in penile injections have not yet been approved by the Food and Drug Administration (FDA) for use in treating impotence. FDA approval usually follows a pharmaceutical company's presentation of the results of clinical trials documenting a particular drug's safety and effectiveness for a specific application. Drugs presented to the FDA are usually new and patent-protected for several years (to ensure a company has the opportunity to recoup its research expense and make a profit). FDA trials are expensive and demanding. Papaverine and phentolamine are not new (although they *are* new in the treatment of impotence) and the patent protection for them has lapsed.

Several pharmaceutical companies have invested the time and money in clinical trials for drugs as they relate to impotence. The one drug presently FDA approved for the treatment of impotence is prostaglandin E1. The FDA protects the consumer by ensuring that a new drug is safe for a particular application. It does not involve itself in the doctor-patient relationship or force a doctor to use a drug for approved applications only. A doctor may suggest a non-FDA-approved treatment option to a patient for a certain medical problem, as long as the patient understands the treatment's usages, risks and benefits. It would put everyone more at ease if papaverine and phentolamine were FDA-approved for the treatment of impotence, but this approval does not now exist.

In addition to the approximately 100,000 American men who use penile shots to treat their impotence, another estimated 500,000 men outside the United States also rely on self-injection therapy. As more drugs are found to be useful, self-injection will undoubtedly become an increasingly common treatment for the impotent male.

psychological factors were contributing to their sexual problems. I did not feel they needed sex therapy, and they concurred. The Perkinses later gave me permission to review taped interviews in which they discussed their experience with impotence, and to comment on their experience and history.

If all couples who faced a problem with impotence were as well-adjusted as Norm and Gloria Perkins, there wouldn't be any need for sex therapists. Remarkably, Norm's bout with alcoholism and a long period of repeated sexual frustration seem to have taken no long-lasting toll on their relationship. Although these problems did cause this couple considerable distress, their crisis brought them closer together in the long run.

Norm's confusion, as well as their attempts to trace his impotence to a familiar factor in their lives — stress, different work schedules, Norm's back pain, their adjustment to Gloria's own reproductive maladies — is a frequent response by couples when the man begins having erectile difficulties. All of these hypotheses are reasonable, given the couple's level of information.

The Perkinses strongly desired to resolve for themselves a problem whose origin they considered psychological. But, since Norm's problem had a physical origin, their heroic efforts to have intercourse twice a week over a seven-year period were doomed to failure. Their marriage temporarily suffered, as Norm admits. A consistent record of dismal lovemaking will have repercussions for even the most well-adjusted couples.

Norm isn't unusual in citing his impotence as the stimulus for his alcoholism. Other parts of this book have outlined the psychological burden of men suffering from impotence, especially over a long period of time. Men with longstanding erectile difficulties often turn to drugs or alcohol for escape from the painful complex of feelings associated with their perceived inadequacy. Substance abuse, however, only postpones the inevitable necessity of facing the problem if the relationship is to survive. Norm realized that his drinking was only adding one more destructive element to his emotional straits. To his credit, he sought help and overcame his problem.

Intuitively, Norm knew that none of the factors that he successively blamed for his problem was truly at fault. As each problem was resolved, his impotence remained. His dogged search for something to blame led him to think that his drinking might be responsible for his difficulties. (In some cases, drinking can be a factor in erectile insufficiency, but Norm's problems existed before his alcoholism.) Later, he concluded that his herniated discs might be interfering with nerves that affected his erectile response. A conversation with his sister during his convalescence from back surgery initiated a chain of events that culminated in his successful treatment.

The inner resources of a couple like Norm and Gloria, their obvious commitment to marriage and family, played a large role in sustaining them during the period of Norm's impotence. Their relationship, despite its hardships, was more important to them than sex per se. Within a few weeks of Norm's successful treatment with injections, they managed to overcome years of suffering, easily adjusting to Norm's injections, quickly putting their family life in order.

Norm's story of the old lady and the still emphasizes how his values put the relatively minor drawbacks of injections in perspective: Whatever inconveniences or reservations he might have had about self-injections were easily outweighed by the treatment's benefits. He's typical of most patients who receive injection treatment for organic impotence. The vast majority of patients who depend on injection therapy adjust easily, without the necessity of consulting an outside therapist.

CHAPTER 7

Ted—
The Implant Option

In this chapter, Ted Englander (not his real name), a fifty-four-year-old, married businessman at the time of his first visit to the clinic in 1988, talks about how a penile implant changed his life. If the decision is carefully considered, an implant may be a highly successful, appropriate therapy. Unlike other choices of treatment, however, it is not reversible.

Ted's Story

Sarah and I met in our sophomore year in college back in 1953. I was busy dating as many girls as I could when I met Sarah. I was a superjock and superstudent rolled into one, or so I thought. Sarah was the kind of girl I could eventually settle down with, but at the time I was far from ready to settle down with anyone. We dated for a while and sex was great—I mean really great.

I lived in a wild football fraternity, and we were always doing crazy things. Sarah once masturbated me with her foot in the school library! We broke up in the summer and I went with someone else. Two years later, in our senior year, Sarah and I got back together. That spring break, we went to Fort Lauderdale: Life felt good to us. We've been monogamous ever since.

After college, Sarah and I got married. I went to business school while Sarah taught second grade. Our sex life was still healthy, although I would fall asleep sometimes after working hard all day, or I'd tell Sarah not to start teasing me because I had to study. Our best times were vacations, when we could both leave the books and papers behind and make love several times a day—wedded bliss!

The kids were born, and I tried to spend time with them, so my work at home each evening started later and later. Try squeezing sex in when you work late, your supermom wife falls asleep early, and four kids jump in your bed in the morning. Sarah and I made love a couple of times a week if we were lucky.

Then the revolution—the kids got bigger and started sleeping late. Sarah and I could stay in bed on the weekends and enjoy each other. But, things weren't quite as enjoyable as they had been. I was nervous about work—whether or not I was going to be promoted to store manager—and Sarah had to play with me a lot to make my erections firm enough for penetration.

Then our oldest, Jeremy, started college. With four kids to put through school, the pressure was on. I needed more and more stimulation for successful sex, but Sarah was understanding and never complained. I started feeling guilty because Sarah had gone from multiple orgasms to one unless we had long foreplay. I felt very insecure about my progressive "loss of manhood," and I wondered what my college buddies would think if they knew about my problem. I devoted more and more time to work and to my children and spent less and less time alone with Sarah.

When our last child, Rob, graduated from college three years ago, the money pressure was finally off. He had a fellowship for graduate school, the other boys were doing well, and our daughter, Liz, had married a lawyer. I was now vice-president of a local retail chain, and Sarah had gone back to work. We went on a three-week vacation alone, the first in years, and sex was a little better. As long as we didn't change positions—I stayed on the bottom—I could perform, but I started to think that maybe my problem wasn't all in my head.

HIGH BLOOD PRESSURE, OVERWEIGHT

When we returned home to New Hampshire, I called my family doctor and scheduled a checkup. I found out I had high blood pressure. Since it had been years since my last checkup, my doctor said I might have had hypertension for years. I had given up smoking when Liz was born, but the doctor said that now I had to give up the rich desserts I loved too. I was forty pounds overweight—me, the last of the great college jocks. I knew I disliked doctors for a reason. Of course, the only football I had played lately was armchair football watching the tube. I went home to give Sarah the "good news"—no more fried foods, no more whipped cream.

As my confidence about sex had decreased, I realized, I had placed more and more emphasis on food and eating. Now, looking back, I realize that as Sarah started feeling guilty that maybe she was responsible for my sagging sex organ, she had made her meals more elaborate. If we finished dinner late and went to bed stuffed, we would both be too "satisfied" and too full to contemplate sex.

So now I was on a diet. Sarah went to the bookstore and bought books about controlling high blood pressure through diet. To make matters worse, my doctor put me on a blood-pressure medication that caused me to lose all desire for sex. He switched medications when I told him I had no sex drive.

I lost weight and felt better—but it was hard to feel good about myself when our sex life had become nonexistent.

Sarah had become quieter, and I was wondering if her teaching was really using up all her energy. I knew Sarah couldn't be unfaithful —or did I? We didn't seem to be talking about anything anymore except my diet!

I lost thirty pounds over seven months. My blood pressure was under control, my retirement was approaching, I had two beautiful grandsons, and everything was great—or so it seemed to outsiders. No one knew Sarah and I were having sex problems because I seemed fine among family and friends. Soon enough I would have time on my hands, I thought, and I wanted to be able to chase Sarah around the house like in the old days. I was afraid to ask Sarah if she even wanted to be chased.

SEX THERAPY

I got up my nerve and called for an appointment with my family doctor. He examined me and checked my testosterone level, which was normal. The doctor could find nothing else obviously wrong with me. He gave me the name of a psychologist who specializes in sex therapy and insisted that I would do better to bring Sarah along. That was the hardest thing I ever had to do—admit I was scared, unhappy, insecure and guilty about sex, or lack of it. Sarah and I had a long talk. It turned out Sarah had the same feelings, but she wasn't sure she really wanted to have sex again. She could under-stand that I wanted to be able to have sex, but she thought it was silly that I didn't feel like a man because I couldn't perform.

To make a long story short, we started seeing the sex therapist. [The Englanders' sex therapist was not Dr. Alma Dell Smith.] I don't know which one of us was more nervous. The therapist forced us to really talk about our problem. Sarah had gotten to the point where she was afraid of sex. Her vagina had gotten very dry with age and lack of use, and she was sure she would split in two if we had sex again. But she desperately wanted to be held and caressed—some-thing I was uncomfortable doing for fear of starting something I couldn't finish.

The therapist explained that sex did not necessarily mean inter-course. She said we should talk about our feelings while we were lying in bed, and we should touch each other all over. She told Sarah not to be afraid to touch my penis, because even if I could get only partially hard, I could still ejaculate and feel good. I could mastur-bate Sarah or play with her breasts or whatever made her feel good. We were given a series of relaxation exercises to practice routinely.

After six months of sex therapy, Sarah and I were finally able to talk easily about our frustrations and fears, but we weren't happy. Sarah was no longer fearful of "real sex" because her vagina had become more lubricated as a result of the exercises we were doing. The therapist had showed Sarah that her guilt feelings were un-founded, that she was not a failure as a wife and shouldn't be shy about expressing her feelings.

Sarah explained that she enjoyed my holding her, but once I started playing with her, she couldn't feel totally satisfied without making love "normally." She wasn't any more comfortable than I was with the "sex-without-intercourse" approach. She wanted to either go all the way or just be held. And I was miserable because I still wanted to be able to "do it."

SOMETHING MORE

I called our sex therapist and told her we needed something more. She told me about Dr. Goldstein, a urologist in Boston who special-ized in impotence treatment.

I came home from work that night feeling better than I had in a long time. I told Sarah about my conversation with the therapist. At least I could now talk to her about my impotence. I told her to make plans to visit Boston and to let our son Jeremy know we would be staying with him one weekend soon. I felt like a four-year-old waiting for Santa Claus instead of a fifty-four-year-old waiting to see a doctor.

Actually, my dislike of doctors in general, and my fear that Dr. Goldstein wouldn't be able to help, increased just as my anticipa-tion of a normal sex life increased. I was driving Sarah crazy.

I haven't spoken enough about my wife. Sarah, despite her own fears, frustrations and anger, is my anchor. She has always been sup-portive of me and never (consciously, at least) made me feel less a man. She went through sex therapy at my request, even though I know she felt very awkward talking openly about sex. Her depres-sions have been reflections of mine, not vice versa. And, despite the changes in our physical relationship, I love Sarah more than ever. I wondered, was it too late to have the romantic vacation we had always dreamed of?

IT'S BASICALLY PHYSICAL

Sarah and I visited Jeremy that fall without telling the family the real reason for our trip to Boston. Dr. Goldstein met with us, asked a lot of questions, examined me and ran some tests, including one called a DICC [see box, page 102], which he said was extremely important. From the DICC, he determined that I had blood storage problems as well as blockages of blood flow to my penis. He explained that whatever anxiety I had felt in the past about my work or my sexual abilities might have hampered my ability to perform, but that my impotence was *basically physical*. Boy, did that take away a load of guilt and worry from Sarah's and my shoulders. I didn't feel great about being impotent, but if there was something physically wrong with me, maybe the doctor could fix it.

Dr. Goldstein explained about the different therapy options. He talked about bypass surgery and explained why it was not a logical option because of my history of high blood pressure and the multiple locations of my circulatory abnormalities. He said there was an injection therapy that a lot of people use successfully and advised me to try it.

INJECTION THERAPY

On our next "visit to Jeremy," Dr. Goldstein gave me a test dose of the papaverine and phentolamine by penile injection [see chapter 6]. I got almost no response. I went back to the office the next day and received a stronger dose.

It's a good thing we were staying in a hotel and not with Jeremy this trip, or my grandchildren would have been treated to an earful. I was like a little boy with a new toy, but it didn't last long. Sarah stripped and I tried to stuff my penis into her vagina. My penis went almost limp, and I wanted to cry in frustration.

Back I went to Dr. Goldstein's office. He made the medicine stronger and again injected my penis. Would I be able to give myself injections? On the way back to the hotel, I could feel Venus rising, and I felt really good about myself.

Sarah had stayed in the hotel, and when I opened the door, my wife was in a startlingly sexy nightgown. I pulled off my clothes confidently and practically pushed Sarah onto the bed. I climbed on top of her. Now that I think about it, there was nothing tender or loving about that moment. There was no foreplay. I was in such a hurry to make love that poor Sarah was almost screaming in pain.

Sarah's tight, unlubricated vagina did nothing for my semierection, as I realized with distress that that was what I had. Sex, once again, was the horror show I had been afraid it would be — for both of us. Neither of us was satisfied physically, and at this point, each day was getting more frustrating.

Once again, I went back to Dr. Goldstein with my tale of woe. Could we pump the dosage way up . . . please? Dr. Goldstein gave me the bad news — the drug therapy wasn't working. I wasn't really interested in using a vacuum device, so the only reasonable alternative was a penile implant.

IMPLANT SURGERY

Dr. Goldstein explained about the different types of implants. This surgery was highly successful, he said, and would enable me to achieve a rigid erection. Wow — I'll do it! Somehow the thought of a real sex life again got me over my lifelong fear of doctors and surgery. Curing my impotence had become my priority.

Dr. Goldstein gave me the opportunity to speak with two of his patients who had had implants put in the year before. They explained how the surgery had changed their lives. They were essentially just like me, with no ability for intercourse before the surgery, and every capability now.

One man mentioned that his erection was shorter now with the implant than it had been before, but my feeling is, better a shorter, functioning erection than a longer, non-functioning one. They also talked about how the implants had affected their wives. One patient said his wife had a hard time adjusting to having sex again and would still prefer not to have vaginal sex, but that he was glad he had had the surgery because now he felt like a man again.

No one had had any physical problems with the implant. They both highly recommended my having the surgery, although I don't think I really needed to be convinced.

When Sarah and I drove to Boston for my surgery, we told the kids I was having prostate surgery and that the urologist in Boston had been highly recommended. Knowing my paranoia about doctors, the kids understood about my wanting to go to "the best."

Dr. Goldstein implanted a three-piece hydraulic device. [*Hydraulic* and *nonhydraulic* implants are discussed starting on page 133 and are shown in the illustrations on pages 134 and 136.] I learned to activate the implant three weeks after my surgery, but he told me to wait another three weeks before having intercourse to allow for complete healing. Try waiting six weeks after surgery for your first successful intercourse in years — talk about impatience! Sarah and I were planning our re-entry into the sexual world, and I realized Sarah was almost as excited as I was. I finally had the proper equipment.

We had figured out from our experience with injection therapy that Sarah's vagina was no longer able to accommodate my penis without discomfort for her. Dr. Goldstein suggested a good lubricant, which Sarah bought. And, from sex therapy, I remembered the importance of foreplay.

Forty-two days after surgery, Sarah set the dining-room table with our best china, lit candles, floated in wearing a sexy negligee and served escargots. We ate slowly. Then, as Sarah cleared the dishes for the next course, I followed her into the kitchen. I will always remember the moment. She was bending over the kitchen sink, and I could feel my slight arousal. Even if I couldn't perform without help, I could still feel. I reached down and pumped the fluid from the reservoir of the implant into the cylinders. Voilà! Instant erection. I reached my arms around Sarah's waist and rubbed my new-found erection against her backside. Sarah told me later that she got wet just feeling me like that–it had been so long.

Our duck à l'orange dried out sitting in the oven, but it was worth it. I carried Sarah to our bedroom.She had the lubricant sitting on the night table. I had always known Sarah was brilliant! We touched each other all over, slowly and gently at first, then more fervently. We used the lubricant on each other as part of our foreplay. I entered Sarah slowly, remembering her discomfort at the hotel in Boston with a much smaller erection. It felt *so* good even though I was still somewhat sore. I ejaculated quickly, but with the firm erection from my implant, I was able to continue intercourse until Sarah had a strong orgasm.

PERPETUAL HONEYMOON

That was eleven months ago. I retired at the age of fifty-five. Sarah had stopped teaching the year before, when her school closed. We took the second honeymoon we had always dreamed of. Sex every day? Sometimes it was twice.

We returned home to more normal lives, but since we're both retired, no one knows what we do all day. Who says no sex after fifty?

Sarah and I bought a time-share vacation home in the Virgin Islands for our perpetual honeymoon. I no longer have any physical discomfort from my surgery, and Sarah loves to tease me by starting to pump my implant for me. I guess we don't have any mental hang-ups about that. I think we're in our second romance and loving it. And pleasure? Only the birth our first granddaughter comes near.

The self confidence that now permeates my being has given me the backbone to meet new people. Dr. Goldstein asked if I would be willing to speak with prospective implant patients, to help others as I was helped.

I'm sure some of our new friends have the same problem I once had. That felt good, to say "once had." Sarah sends her love—from the bedroom.

Dr. Irwin Goldstein: The Medical Perspective

Penile implants, or *penile prostheses,* as they are known in medical terms, are devices that a urologist surgically inserts into the corpora cavernosa (erection chambers) of the patient's penis (see illustrations, pages 134 and 136). One way or another, these devices re-create stiffness in the penis, which the patient's own disabled erectile physiology can no longer provide.

Implants are one of impotence therapy's dazzling success stories. They are the most reliable therapy available for restoring erections, which gives them an enormous emotional appeal. For the man who doesn't want to use injection therapy and whose vascular blockages are too numerous and diffuse to benefit from reconstructive surgery, they are usually the best alternative. But, unlike the other treatments we've discussed, implants injure what's left of the man's own erectile system, and are therefore considered irreversible.

The patient who is contemplating implant surgery should understand that an erection with an implant may not look or feel exactly like his old erections. Often, a session or more with a knowledgeable sex therapist is the easiest way of making the transition to lovemaking after implant surgery. The therapist can suggest subtle adjustments in technique for enabling the patient and his partner to achieve maximum satisfaction. I recommend sex therapy more and more frequently to my patients. Urologists and therapists are coming to recognize that patients' problems, even if they are primarily medical, are not devoid of secondary psychological reactions. Both problems need attention. As I hope the case histories in this book demonstrate, the mind-body connection in sexual function is very important.

The success of this kind of surgery depends on matching patient expectations with the reality of what an implant can actually accomplish. For Ted Englander and his wife, expectations were met.

A BRIEF HISTORY OF IMPLANTS

Surgeons began their first efforts with penile implants in the 1930s and 1940s as a way of helping men whose penises had been seriously damaged by trauma (injury), often the result of an auto accident or of military combat.

It's possible these surgeons took their inspiration from the animal world. As I mentioned in chapter 2, many mammals have a bone inside the penis that assists in the erectile process. Surgeons hoping to create a "human penile bone" turned to the closest logical source for their material, the patients themselves. Thus, the first implants were fashioned from cartilage taken from the patient's own ribs.

The use of the patient's own rib cartilage minimized the likelihood of his immune system's rejecting the implant, but other problems prevented the procedure from ever becoming a practical solution for impotence. Chest surgery can be risky, and ribs and penises are rarely the same size and shape. Even when a surgeon found a rib that fit, he couldn't guarantee long-term results; in many patients the cartilage implant weakened or disappeared entirely, absorbed into the patient's own body.

The evolution from cartilage implants to the first reliable modern implant in the early 1970s involved almost two decades of research with various materials and implantation techniques.

Implants need to be flexible without being fragile. And they need to be "inert," meaning the implant material won't provoke a reaction in sensitive penile tissue. Acrylic was tried and rejected—too brittle, and some patients had bad reactions. Polyethylene came next, which was a slight improvement. But, the unqualified success was silicone. Silicone rods are both durable and flexible, so flexible they can be bent almost double without breaking. Silicone, along with the even more recent innovation, polyurethane, continues to be the material of choice for most implant manufacturers.

Almost as important, it came to be understood that implants worked best if placed *inside* the penis's corpora cavernosa (the erection chambers). For the most part, until the late 1950s they had been implanted under the skin of the penis, *outside* the erection chambers.

In 1973, the first series of inert silicone implants was reported in the medical literature. These implants proved to be highly effective. Since the successes of the early 1970s, steady improvements have been made in implant design.

Implants are popularly classified as "inflatable" and "noninflatable" models, but I prefer to think of implants as either *hydraulic* or *nonhydraulic*, depending on whether they use solid or fluid-filled cylinders to make the penis rigid.

NONHYDRAULIC IMPLANTS

Nonhydraulic implants (also known as mechanical or semirigid implants) are the simplest type of penile prosthesis. Typically, they

Nonhydraulic Penile Implant

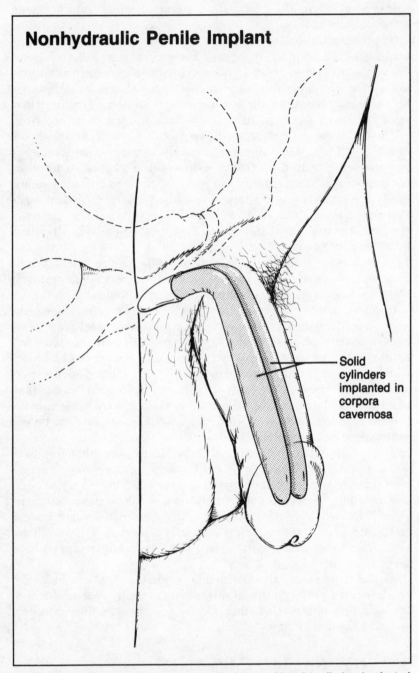

Solid
cylinders
implanted in
corpora
cavernosa

Nonhydraulic penile implants provide penile rigidity with solid cylinders implanted in the corpora cavernosa. Most models keep the penis rigid at all times. Nonhydraulic implants do not increase the circumference of the penis.

consist of a pair of rods inserted into the two large erection chambers of the penis (see illustration, opposite page). With one exception, all models of nonhydraulic implants keep the penis rigid all the time, but there is no increase in the circumference of the penis with any of them. For almost all men, a nonhydraulic implant will make the penis rigid enough for intercourse. Men with unusually long penises, however, may require the rigidity that can be achieved with a three-piece hydraulic implant.

Since nonhydraulic implants have few moving parts, they usually (though not necessarily) have lower failure rates than hydraulic models. They require little or no effort to activate (since in most cases the penis is always rigid enough for intercourse). Their simpler design also means that they require less complicated implantation surgery than do hydraulic prostheses. Depending on the patient and the particular model of nonhydraulic implant, an overnight hospital stay may not even be required. On average, the cost of a nonhydraulic implant and its associated surgical and hospital fees tends to be less than the cost of a hydraulic implant.

Some nonhydraulic implants can present a cosmetic problem because of the penis's constant rigidity. This can be handled by learning how to properly position the penis in the underwear. Still, a man who often finds himself in circumstances where public nudity is required (such as a health-club locker room) may find this embarrassing.

Newer nonhydraulic models make the presence of the implant less apparent to casual observers, regardless of a man's state of dress. They allow the implant to be bent downward, so the penis is positioned like an ordinary flaccid penis. Some implants now have flexible sections, located at the base of the penis, that enable the erection to be bent against the leg. Other models contain a twisted wire core covered with silicone, so the implant may be bent down—and stay down—instead of springing upright when released from underclothing. A newer model even allows for diminished rigidity in the flaccid state. This model consists of silicone segments attached by a wire cable.

HYDRAULIC IMPLANTS

Hydraulic implants are made up of three components—a pair of hollow cylinders placed inside the corpora cavernosa in the penis, a reservoir of fluid (sterile saline solution) and a pump. To make the penis erect, you pump fluid from the reservoir to the cylinders; to make the penis flaccid, the process is reversed.

Hydraulic implants come in three-, two- and one-piece versions, depending on whether the components are configured separately

Hydraulic Penile Implant (Three-Piece Type)

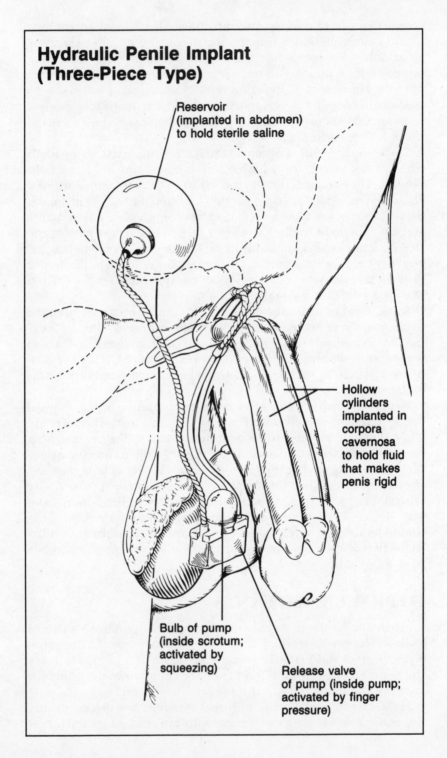

Reservoir (implanted in abdomen) to hold sterile saline

Hollow cylinders implanted in corpora cavernosa to hold fluid that makes penis rigid

Bulb of pump (inside scrotum; activated by squeezing)

Release valve of pump (inside pump; activated by finger pressure)

or together. The three-piece type is shown in the illustration on page 136. In a three-piece implant, the pump is surgically inserted inside the scrotum, between or beside the testicles, the reservoir is positioned in the lower abdomen under the stomach muscles, and the cylinders are inside the erection chambers of the penis.

Three-piece hydraulic implants come closest to mimicking a natural erection. The patient squeezes the pump in his scrotum to transfer fluid from the reservoir to the cylinders in his penis. The circumference of the penis increases as the man continues pumping, and the penis seems to inflate, giving the device its popular name, the "inflatable implant." Ten to twenty squeezes are usually enough to make the flaccid penis wider and rigid. In most cases, there's no significant increase in length during activation. The "erection" looks and feels nearly natural, and is more than adequate for penetration. You return the penis to the flaccid state by pressing a release valve on the scrotal pump. Saline solution in the cylinders flows back to the reservoir, where it is stored. The penis becomes soft and returns to its former circumference. The saline solution simply goes back and forth, from reservoir to cylinders and back, depending on the desired state of erection or flaccidity.

Two-piece hydraulic implants combine the pump and reservoir in a single unit that fits in the scrotum. The combined pump-reservoir is larger than the pump used in a three-piece implant, but it holds less solution than a separate abdominal reservoir. As you might expect, with less fluid to flow into the cavernosal cylinders, the increase in rigidity from the flaccid to the erect state may not be quite so great as with a three-piece unit. In its favor, the two-piece hydraulic implant is simpler to install than the traditional three-piece device.

One-piece hydraulic implants combine pump, reservoir and cylinder into a single slender device. A complete unit is fitted into each corpus cavernosum. Mechanically, the one-piece unit is the simplest of all hydraulic implants. Pressing the end of the implant (behind the glans) pumps fluid into the hollow portion of the

---

Hydraulic penile implants provide penile rigidity by infusing pressurized fluid (sterile saline) into hollow cylinders implanted in the corpora cavernosa. A three-piece type is shown on page 136. In the flaccid state, the saline is primarily in the reservoir, which is surgically placed in the lower abdomen under the stomach muscles. In the erect state, the saline is primarily in the cylinders. The pump, which is placed in the scrotum, controls the location of the saline. Squeezing the bulb of the pump transfers the saline from the reservoir into the cylinders and simulates an erection. Pressing the release valve under the bulb allows the fluid in the cylinders to transfer back into the reservoir and allows the penis to return to a flaccid state. The entire mechanism is implanted under the surface of the skin and is not visible in any way.

cylinder, located in the shaft of the penis. This makes the penis more rigid, but doesn't affect its circumference. One-piece implants usually become sufficiently rigid for penetration, but less rigid than either the two- or three-piece hydraulic implants. In addition, the penis doesn't become quite as flaccid as it does with other hydraulic implants.

Hydraulic implants, especially the three-piece units, have the appeal of nearly duplicating the penis's natural states of flaccidity and erection. Also, the three-piece hydraulic implants (and possibly the two-piece) can give even a long penis enough rigidity for intercourse. The price for this versatility is a higher mechanical failure rate and a higher cost than is found with nonhydraulic implants. Hydraulic implants may also be somewhat more difficult for the man to operate. In general, patients lacking manual dexterity (or a steady partner willing to take responsibility for learning to operate the implant) should consider a nonhydraulic implant.

IMPLANT SURGERY AND RECOVERY

Depending on your state of health, the inclination of your surgeon and the type of implant involved, implant surgery may be performed under general, spinal or local anesthesia. The sites of the incisions in the penis, perineum, abdomen and scrotum also vary according to the implant and the surgeon's preference. In any event, even the three-piece hydraulic implant requires only one skin incision. For a nonhydraulic implant, the surgical procedure usually lasts about an hour; a three-piece hydraulic implant takes an hour and a half to two hours.

After the operation, your penis and scrotum will probably be swollen and tender, and for a day or two you may feel a burning sensation when you urinate. Postoperative pain is variable, but in general you can expect the discomfort to last for four to six weeks. Most patients require narcotic medication for pain control. During this time you will be advised to avoid any heavy lifting, which could strain the groin area.

The body reacts to the components of an implant by encasing them in a thin layer of scar tissue. This is a perfectly natural response. Minimizing excessive scarring, and ensuring that scarring occurs evenly, are two of the reasons why you should closely follow your urologist's suggestions during the period of convalescence. Positioning your penis against your abdomen, holding it in place with an athletic supporter or jockey-style underwear, reduces the chance of uneven scarring that could cause the penis to bend. This is also the most comfortable position for the penis during healing.

With the three-piece hydraulic implant, it is important that scar tissue forms around a full reservoir. In other words, the penis should be kept flaccid (cylinders empty) for at least three to four weeks after surgery. If scar tissue is allowed to form around a partially full reservoir, the reservoir may never expand sufficiently to hold the full volume of fluid in the system. Nor can the cylinders in the shaft drain completely, so the penis never becomes truly flaccid. Waiting three or four weeks for the scarring to complete itself around the reservoir has been found to allow the system to fill and empty completely.

After three or four weeks, I teach all patients how to activate and deactivate their hydraulic implants. The first one or two inflations of the device may be painful, but the implant needs to be activated in order to begin stretching the scar tissue surrounding the shaft cylinders. Any discomfort usually disappears as the tissue stretches and healing progresses.

Most patients, regardless of the type of implant, can resume intercourse six weeks after surgery. This waiting period ensures complete healing and should allow pain-free intercourse. You should wait longer if the implant area is still painful during erection. A water-soluble lubricant applied to the shaft of the penis may reduce any uncomfortable sensitivity around the incision area.

TED ENGLANDER, SENSUOUS GRANDFATHER

Ted Englander and his wife, Sarah, were referred to me by a sex therapist, who described them as a highly motivated couple desiring treatment for impotence.

Ted had been having erection difficulties for three to five years and had a history of cigarette smoking, excess weight and high blood pressure (which was under control). He had a family history of heart disease and a slightly elevated cholesterol level. He was able to achieve only 50 percent of the erection rigidity that he had had as a young adult.

Ted also told me that he could sustain his erection for only a few minutes during masturbation, during intercourse and on awakening in the morning. He and Sarah were, however, still having sex with occasional successful vaginal penetration—especially on vacations.

Their previous efforts in sex therapy had enabled them to reach a remarkable level of communication and openness with respect to their sexual desires and needs. In their excitement to get going on diagnosis and treatment of Ted's impotence, they reminded me of youngsters at the entrance to Disneyland.

A quick check of Ted's penile blood pressure showed that it was abnormally low compared to the blood pressure in his arm. His family doctor had already checked his testosterone level, and it was normal.

In view of Ted's history of consistent erectile changes for a sustained period of time, his lack of erectile improvement with sex therapy and his low penile blood pressure, I was strongly suspicious that Ted had a physical problem—most likely a circulatory abnormality.

The next step was to do a DICC study. The study showed that Ted's penis contained many abnormal areas, resulting in a deficient blood-storage mechanism and insufficient pressure in the arteries of his erection chambers.

Ted chose to try self-injections first. His reason was that this was a reversible method of treatment and one that would not involve surgery—an event he had managed to avoid all his life. Unfortunately, the erections that resulted from the injections were not sufficiently rigid or sustained. Today, Ted would receive a combination of injectable drugs, including papaverine, phentolamine and prostaglandin El. At the time he was treated, prostaglandin El was not available.

He was not a good candidate for penile vascular surgery because of the multiple areas of damage in his storage mechanism.

Ted then decided to consider a penile implant. I reviewed the various implants, and Ted spoke with two implant users. He decided on the three-piece hydraulic model because of its excellent "track record" in this country, and because it simulated a natural erection more closely than any of the other models.

Ted underwent the surgery without any problems and was easily taught to activate and deactivate the pump mechanism. He made sure that Sarah was also capable of operating the device, reminding me that it was "her device as well."

Ted and Sarah were a nearly ideal couple for impotence treatment. They had a long history of marital compatibility and a genuine love for each other.

Sarah, like many older women, was experiencing some sexual problems of her own (the vaginal dryness that Ted refers to), but this difficulty may have increased her understanding of her husband's changing body. In any case, extended foreplay and a lubricant were all that was needed to overcome this particular problem.

As Ted says, he and his wife had no "mental hang-ups" about integrating the implant device into their foreplay and lovemaking. And, while they may be on a "perpetual honeymoon," their expectations of themselves are fundmentally realistic.

Ted was a good candidate for an implant, and Ted and Sarah exemplify couples who are helped by a combination of psychologically oriented sex therapy and surgical treatment for impotence.

QUESTIONS AND ANSWERS
ABOUT IMPLANTS

What are the chances I'll be happy with an implant? Extremely good. Reports vary, but approximately 80 to 90 percent of implant recipients report a high degree of satisfaction with their device. If you're considering an implant, carefully discuss your expectations of the implant with your urologist before the surgery. Postoperative dissatisfaction can almost always be traced to the patient's unfulfilled expectations. If you and your partner understand the reality of implant surgery and adjust your expectations to match that reality, then you stand an excellent chance of restoring your sex life in a satisfactory manner.

Will an implant give me back my erection, just like it used to be? Probably not. Implants do not re-create normal erections. An implant is an artificial device designed to give your penis enough rigidity for you to have intercourse. In most cases, this means the erection from an implant is not as "good" as an erection from a normally functioning penis. None of the implants available today increases the size or firmness of the head of the penis, for example, or of the tissue surrounding the *urethra*, the penis's central passageway for urine and semen. Firmness in both areas aids in penetration and satisfactory intercourse. After implant surgery, enlargement of the glans and urethra still depends on the sexual stimulation that accompanies intercourse.

Most patients also report that the erection produced by an implant is not as long as they remember their normal erections having been. We aren't completely sure why this should be, but part of the answer may be that implants are necessarily installed in flaccid penises. A surgeon is limited to installing implants that he can fit comfortably into the corpora cavernosa of the stretched, but still flaccid, penis. The smooth-muscle tissue of the flaccid penis is constricted. But the smooth-muscle tissue of an aroused penis is relaxed, permitting it to stretch further. A flaccid penis will simply not stretch to be as long as the same penis in a state of erection. This means that the erection from an implant may be as much as one or two inches shorter than the man's previous natural erections.

The circumference of an erection may also be affected by an implant. With a three-piece hydraulic implant, the penis's circumference will increase significantly as the penis becomes erect. But most implants don't have this effect. With most implants, hydraulic or nonhydraulic, there's a good chance the circumference of the rigid penis will be smaller than that of a patient's previous natural erection.

Will an implant bring back my interest in sex? That depends upon whether your lack of interest is connected to an inability to have an erection or upon other factors. As a rule, an implant won't resuscitate a flagging libido (sex drive), except insofar as interest is related to the ability to have an erection sufficient for intercourse. As Dr. Alma Dell Smith points out in chapter 3, arousal involves a complex interplay of psychological factors, most of which are beyond the influence of an implant. If you truly want to have intercourse, but can't, an implant will help restore your sexual appetite. If, on the other hand, you can't have intercourse—and don't really care if you regain the ability or not—it's unlikely an implant will solve the problem.

Will an implant alter the sensation in my penis? Probably not. Implants don't usually interfere with sensation in the penis. After the implant, you should have the same sensations as you did before you had the surgery. If you could achieve orgasm and ejaculate before you had the implant, you can expect to do so after the implant. By the same token, don't expect an implant to bring back those abilities if you lost them prior to surgery. An implant may interfere with ejaculatory ability if you have unresolved psychological issues concerning the procedure. Any event which impinges on the emotional experience of sex has the potential for disrupting orgasm, which is why I counsel my patients to tailor their expectations according to what they may reasonably expect from an implant—not what they might wish it could do.

After the implant surgery, will my penis always be erect? Some implants mimic the penis's natural ability to alternate between states of erection and flaccidity. The realism varies with the specific device. With most nonhydraulic implants, the only difference between these states is the position of the penis—up for "erect," down for "flaccid." Though seemingly minor, this distinction can make quite a difference in appearance when you dress, or if you find yourself in circumstances that entail public nudity. With hydraulic implants, most noticeably the three-piece hydraulic models, the rigidity and circumference of the penis increase dramatically as the penis becomes erect. When flaccid, the same penis is usually indistinguishable from a flaccid penis without an implant.

I've heard that an implant could interfere with my ability to urinate. Is this true? It's rare, but this complication does sometimes occur. Depending on the type of implant, some men notice a change in their urinary ability after the surgery. It's not uncommon during the postoperative period for a man to have difficulty initiating urination, especially if urination is painful. In almost all cases this discomfort soon disappears. Some men report that a few drops of urine dribble from the tip of the penis after they finish urinating. Other men have noticed that their urine seems to flow less forcefully than before surgery, especially with those implants that maintain the penis in a constant state of rigidity. Neither of these conditions is painful. They require little, if any, attention other than patient awareness, and as I said, they're relatively rare.

Will I lose any blood during the surgery? Will I require a blood transfusion? Public awareness of AIDS has increased patients' fears of contracting the disease through a contaminated batch of blood. Implant surgery involves little loss of blood and usually requires no blood transfusions.

What are the possible complications of having an implant? Any surgery that introduces a foreign substance into the body exposes the patient to a small risk of infection (about a 1 to 8 percent chance according to the medical literature). In most cases of infection with an implant, the implant must be surgically removed. There are cases where the implant may be reimplanted within days after removal, but most urologists prefer to wait several weeks to months before considering reimplanting the device.

Mechanical failure is also a risk whenever prosthetic materials and devices are used. Implants sometimes break, or erode through the penis. The offending implant then has to be surgically removed and replaced. The complexity of hydraulic implants causes them to fail more frequently than nonhydraulic ones. The most common problem with hydraulic implants is leakage, which requires that the abnormal component, or if necessary the entire implant, be removed and replaced with a functioning component or device.

What if I change my mind after I have the implant? For example, suppose a few years after I get the implant I want to give penile injections or reconstructive surgery a try—could I have the implant removed? You could have the implant removed. But your chances of success with self-injection therapy or reconstructive surgery would be extremely slim. The only consistently successful treatment in patients who have had implants removed is installation of another implant or reliance on a vacuum constriction device. The nature of implant surgery inevitably causes injury and scarring of the penis's erectile tissue. Treatments like self-injection or reconstructive surgery depend on this tissue's being virtually intact. Removing the implant doesn't restore erectile tissue to its state before the surgery. Try other treatments, when appropriate, before electing to have an implant.

Does health insurance normally cover implant surgery? Insurance plans and health maintenance organizations vary widely in their coverage of treatment for impotence. Check with your insurance company or HMO (health maintenance organization) for details concerning your coverage.

Dr. Alma Dell Smith—
The Psychological Perspective

I was not involved in the Englanders' therapy, although, with their permission, I did review and comment on their history based on their taped interviews and my discussions with Dr. Goldstein. The therapy they did have before seeing Dr. Goldstein made it easier for them to discuss their fears and frustrations and to make the decision ultimately to go ahead with the implant surgery.

———— ◆ ————

Most implant users adjust easily to the device and do well, but a minority of men—and sometimes their partners—find they are dissatisfied with their implants. For example:

1. Men and their sex partners who are preoccupied with the size of the penis may be unhappy with the penis's appearance after the implant has been inserted, and this in turn can affect their sexual appetite and performance.

2. Men who ejaculate very quickly during intercourse may dislike being asked by their partners to continue intercourse after ejaculation. With an implant, it is possible for a man to continue indefinitely, but some men dislike doing so.

3. Men who are not accustomed to—or who dislike—foreplay may attempt intercourse with an implant without first being sexually aroused. They may then find that they do not achieve orgasm.

4. Couples who are not open to variation in sexual positions and techniques may continue in an old "style" that is not well adapted to the implant.

5. Patients who have been coerced into surgery with the threat of a partner's leaving or seeking sexual satisfaction elsewhere have a predictably poor sexual adjustment after implant surgery.

———— ◆ ————

Sex therapy is helpful in almost any impotence treatment plan, but is particularly so prior to and after penile implant surgery. Such therapy may include helping patients to focus less on erectile performance and more on the entire process of lovemaking, including caressing, foreplay and fantasy. To this end, *sensate focus exercises* (see chapter 3, pages 45 and 49), in which partners give pleasure to each other without intercourse, are encouraged. When Ted and Sarah Englander undertook these exercises, they were able to communicate their feelings more clearly than they had in years.

Fears and expectations of the patient and his partner need to be brought into the open for discussion. Brief marital counseling may be important to allow both people to express their feelings and fears about the surgery, the new "equipment" and the new capabilities. Sarah, for example, was concerned that Ted would make excessive sexual demands on her once he had the implant.

I like to think of sex therapy for implant patients as the same as the physical rehabilitation prescribed for patients undergoing cardiac or orthopedic surgery. Even three or four sessions can make the difference between a good sexual adjustment and a poor one.

CHAPTER 8

Special Concerns

- **Diabetes**
- **Peyronie's Disease**
- **Spinal-Cord Injuries and Other Neurologic Disorders**
- **Low Testosterone and Other Hormonal Disorders**
- **Priapism**
- **Cancer**
- **Impotence in Teenagers and the Elderly**
- **Medication-Associated Impotence**

In the previous four chapters I've focused primarily on two major causes of organic impotence—pelvic injury, which can cause scarring of the blood vessels and erectile tissues; and atherosclerosis—fatty deposits in the blood vessels—which can cause circulatory abnormalities in and around the penis. We've also discussed psychogenic impotence (see chapter 3).

A broad range of other medical conditions and circumstances can also influence potency. Conditions like diabetes, Peyronie's disease, spinal-cord injuries and other neurologic problems, low testosterone, priapism, cancer, aging and certain medications can also affect erectile functioning.

Until recently, medicine's preoccupation with the life-threatening effects of certain diseases didn't allow doctors to devote much attention to their effects on a man's love life. Happily, that situation is changing. Though treatment in many cases is far from perfect, we continue to make progress, and rarely are patients left, as they once were, without options for restored potency.

DIABETES MELLITUS

Diabetes mellitus is a disorder of carbohydrate metabolism associated with high blood glucose (sugar) levels. It is caused in some cases by the failure of the pancreas to produce enough of the hormone *insulin*. It represents one group of medical disorders most frequently associated with erection problems. Studies have shown that approximately 50 percent of men with diabetes mellitus will develop impotence. In real numbers, this means that impotence is a problem for over two million diabetic men in the United States.

In the *nondiabetic* population, approximately 3 percent of forty-year-old men are impotent; by age sixty, the percentage of impotent men increases to 20 percent. The largest part of the increase in non-diabetics occurs in men after age fifty. In diabetics, the likelihood of impotence occurs at an even earlier age, with the largest increase happening in men after age forty. By age forty-five, better than a quarter of diabetic men are impotent.

Impotence may occur regardless of the type of treatment the diabetic man receives — that is, whether the disease is treated with injectable insulin or oral medication. It may occur early or late in the course of the disease, although the risk of developing impotence seems to increase with the duration of the diabetes. Occasionally, impotence is the first sign of diabetes.

It is possible that better management of the diabetic patient, with stricter control of blood glucose, could result in a decline in impotence among diabetics, but thus far there's no evidence to support this.

Much research is being performed to understand why patients with diabetes develop impotence. At the present time, researchers have discovered damage in the relaxation nerves that are involved in the erection process, and in the endothelial cells that line the spaces in the erectile tissue (see illustration, page 13). Both these kinds of damage affect the relaxation of smooth muscle, a factor critical to the erection process.

———— ♦ ————

Most urologists take a conservative approach to treating impotence in diabetics, emphasizing behaviorally oriented sex therapy (see chapter 3), vacuum constriction devices (see box, page 169) or self-injection therapy (see chapter 6). Diabetics are not usually good candidates for reconstructive surgery on their penile arteries and veins because they often have multiple problems with the nerves, cells lining the erectile spaces, erectile tissue and blood vessels throughout the entire penis.

Many diabetics opt for penile implants. It's not uncommon for as much as a third of some urologists'implant patients to be diabetic. The vast majority of diabetics report excellent restoration of their erectile function after an implant.

Many of my own patients are diabetic. Two in particular deserve special mention.

Several years ago I was invited to speak about new methods of diagnosis and treatment of impotence on a call-in radio show. John, the show's fifty-year-old producer, approached me after the show, as I was preparing to leave. He informed me that he had enjoyed the show and was fascinated by the new information. He was especially interested in the enthusiastic response by listeners who had telephoned into the program.

John told me that he himself had been a diabetic and dependent on injectable insulin for several years. In the last two years he had started having erection problems. He hadn't had intercourse in over a year. He thought his impotence was the result of his diabetes but wasn't completely sure. Until the radio show, he'd assumed that nothing could be done for him; impotence, like his diabetes, was just something he'd have to accept. This didn't surprise me. I've often found that men with longstanding medical problems often assume, without consulting their physicians, that "secondary" problems like impotence aren't treatable.

I assured John that almost all impotence is treatable and encouraged him to come to the clinic. John underwent the usual full evaluation—with the exception that the clinic staff treated him like a broadcasting celebrity. We discovered he had extensive blockages in his penile arteries, nerve damage and a compromised storage mechanism. He tried injection therapy, but it wasn't that successful. After we arranged for him to speak with several patients who had had penile implants, he finally decided to undergo implant surgery himself.

John selected a nonhydraulic implant. The device he chose is composed of two cylinders made out of silicone segments strung along a cable, much like beads on a string. One cylinder is implanted in each corpus cavernosum. When the patient pushes the top of the penis down toward the groin, the cable tightens, pulling the sections together. This produces an erection of excellent rigidity. After intercourse, the patient releases the cable. No longer bound closely together, the sections then allow the penis to mimic a flaccid state.

This implant is the first and only nonhydraulic type to offer the patient a choice between rigid and flaccid states. Previously, only hydraulic devices could provide patients with this capability (see chapter 7).

John underwent the surgery with great excitement. His friends at the radio station were entirely supportive. John was delighted with his new capability. During visits to the clinic to learn how to activate the implant, he reported feeling more outgoing and confident. His radio friends nicknamed him "Superman." He sent a letter to the office thanking everyone and describing a recent vacation he took with his wife. During a follow-up to the radio program, John accompanied me and discussed his experience on the air.

———— ♦ ————

Alan, another of my diabetic patients, was a forty-three-year-old computer engineer when he came to see me. As fellow engineers, we hit it off from his first visit in the fall of 1987.

Alan's examination showed that his penile arteries and nerves were working fine (in contrast to John's and those of most diabetics), but he had some problems with his storage mechanism. After we discussed various treatment possibilities, Alan decided he wanted to try surgery to restore his storage mechanism. Alan's diabetes would normally have dissuaded me from performing reconstructive surgery—the accounts of other urologists who had tried reconstructive surgery in diabetics were not encouraging. I convinced Alan to at least try self-injection therapy first.

The penile injections made a vast improvement in Alan's erections, but, as a single man, he didn't feel comfortable with the necessity of injecting himself before having intercourse. He continued to press me for surgery, hoping that it would restore his own natural function. At the time, he ruled out any consideration of an implant. In the end, my worries about the poor results reported by other surgeons were offset by Alan's lack of artery or nerve problems, and I went ahead with the surgery.

The initial results of Alan's surgery were exciting—for the first time in a year he was waking up with rigid erections. But, within three months, his erections began losing their rigidity, and after six months he lost most of the improvement. A follow-up DICC study showed virtually no improvement in his storage mechanism.

We have at the present time stopped performing reconstructive surgery for most diabetics because of the research findings demonstrating diffuse nerve and blood-vessel damage with this disease, neither of which can be helped by surgery.

Today, Alan is again using penile injections, with good results. He would reconsider a further reconstructive procedure if we felt it would be successful. He calls the office every six months or so for follow-up information on state-of-the-art developments.

Much additional research needs to be done to increase our understanding of the exact nature of erectile dysfunction in diabetes. In the meantime, other treatment options such as penile implants, penile injections or vacuum constriction devices can enable nearly all diabetic men to enjoy a satisfying love life.

PEYRONIE'S DISEASE

In 1773 François de la Peyronie, physician to Louis XIV, described the presence of a hard, nodular *plaque* (area of localized tissue hardness) in a patient's penis. The plaque was located just under the skin, on the top part of the penile shaft. The patient's penis also made a sharp upward bend during erection. Peyronie erroneously believed that the plaque was the result of a venereal infection. He recommended first eradicating the infection, and then treating the plaque by having the patient bathe in a river located in the nearby Pyrenees.

The distinctive curvature of the erection in men with *Peyronie's disease* results from an area of scarring in the tunica (see illustration, page 152). Imagine a long balloon, deflated, with a piece of tape on one side. The wall of the balloon loses its elasticity in the area where it comes in contact with the tape. If you inflate the balloon, it will bend in the direction of the tape.

Scarring, like tape on the balloon, makes the tunica stiff in one area on one side of the penis. The tunica on the opposite side of the penis remains elastic. As the penis becomes erect, it bends in the direction of the scar.

The incidence of Peyronie's disease is difficult to identify, but approximately 1 percent of a population of men between ages thirty and sixty-five were found to have this condition. More than 90 percent of all cases of Peyronie's disease occur between ages forty and seventy years.

The true origin of Peyronie's disease is unclear. It appears to be associated with the formation of fibrous tissue at the site of an injury to the penis. The tendency to form this kind of fibrous scar tissue may be inherited.

Studies of penile tissue from patients in the early stages of Peyronie's disease show the presence of inflammation under the *tunica albuginea*, the fibrous coat surrounding the erectile tissue. Similar studies of tissues taken from patients in later stages of the disease show dense fibrous formation and in some cases deposits of calcium and even bone in these plaque areas. With some patients,

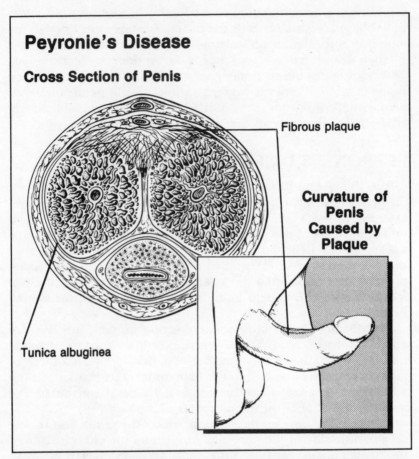

Peyronie's Disease

Cross Section of Penis

Fibrous plaque

Curvature of Penis Caused by Plaque

Tunica albuginea

Peyronie's disease involves the scarring of a region of the tunica (fibrous coat) of the erection chamber(s) and the formation of a hard, nodular plaque in the scarred area, which is most commonly on the top part of the penis, just under the skin. Peyronie's disease may result in a bending of the erection toward the scarred, fibrous plaque because the plaque resists expansion while the rest of the fibrous coat, being elastic, allows for expansion.

extensive scarring extends from the tunica to involve the erectile tissue, which then can no longer expand and compress the subtunical space. The patient's storage mechanism may thus be undermined.

Most cases of Peyronie's disease occur in men in their thirties and forties, but there have been reports of teenage patients as well as men in their eighties with this condition. The four main symptoms of Peyronie's disease are: presence of a plaque, curvature of the erection, painful intercourse (either because the erection itself is painful or because it hurts the partner) and erectile problems. Plaques are usually the size of thumbnails, but may be smaller or much larger. The erection usually curves upward, but variation sometimes occurs here too, with the erection bending to either side or downward.

In medical parlance, Peyronie's disease is called "self-limiting," meaning the process eventually stops without treatment. Its sufferers are then left with varying degrees of scarring of the tunica, which may then result in erectile problems.

The progression of Peyronie's disease varies from patient to patient. Many patients with a minor curvature of the erection, and full potency, report gradual improvement in the curvature without any treatment at all. This may be because the areas of scarring of the tunica soften up, restoring some of the tunica's lost elasticity.

An alternative mechanism in some patients' improvement is that the scarring becomes *more* extensive, involving both sides of each erection chamber of the penis, thus eliminating the inclination of the erection to curve.

Some patients are left with a marked deformity, often associated with pain. Such patients tend to diminish their sexual activity. But, then, as sexual activity declines, their pain and curvature begin to decrease.

Treatment of Peyronie's disease requires weighing the benefits of a potential remedy against its potential complications. Some treatments may pose risks for the erection process itself. Common treatments include: use of vitamin E (as a topical ointment or taken orally or both); use of oral medication called *paraminobenzoate*; radiation; enzymes called *collagenases*; *steroids* (anti-inflammatory medications); and ultrasound treatments. Several surgical treatments have evolved for Peyronie's disease: excision of the plaque, then filling in the resulting space with artificial graft material or skin grafts; removal of a segment of tunica on the side of the penis opposite the plaque, thereby compensating for the bend; or placement of a penile implant. The decision to have any of these procedures depends on the size of the plaque, the degree of curvature and how well the patient's own erectile process still functions.

———— ♦ ————

Richard, a forty-four-year-old electrical lineman, is typical of many of my patients with Peyronie's disease. For two months before visiting the clinic, he'd felt pain in the shaft of his penis during erections. The discomfort was minimal when his penis was flaccid, but over eight weeks the pain had become excruciating in his erections. As the pain increased, he and his wife had intercourse less frequently, and for far shorter periods of time. Richard's erections curved slightly upward and to the left, but there wasn't any obvious change in the rigidity of his erections.

Richard's penis had a hard nodule on the top part of the shaft. After diagnosing his Peyronie's disease, I prescribed oral and topical vitamin E, oral anti-inflammatory medications and a painkiller. He was also instructed to photograph his erections in order to document any changes in the curvature.

After six months, Richard's pain decreased, but his curvature worsened. He was able to have intercourse, but the rigidity and sustaining capability of his erections were diminishing. A year after his initial visit, the Peyronie's disease stabilized and he stopped taking all medication because he noted little improvement. A DICC study showed erection problems with blood-storage abnormalities at the site of his curvature.

We discussed several treatment options. Richard initially decided to take a wait-and-see attitude, but as another six months went by, intercourse became more and more difficult for him. Neither curvature nor pain were the problem; he simply couldn't sustain his erections for very long. Penile injections provided him with moderate improvement in his erections, although there was some initial difficulty injecting around the plaque. He continues to use self-injection therapy, although he's now considering an implant because his erectile sustaining capability is declining even with a combination of papaverine, phentolamine and prostaglandin E1.

SPINAL-CORD INJURIES AND OTHER NEUROLOGIC DISORDERS

Neurological disorders may be divided into those that affect the *central nervous system* (the brain and spinal cord) and those that affect the *peripheral nervous system* (the *sensory* and *motor* nerves that run between the brain and spinal cord and the rest of the body, and control sensation and movement).

Parkinson's disease, Alzheimer's disease, multiple sclerosis and spinal-cord injury are four examples, out of dozens, that involve the brain and spinal cord. Diabetes, lead poisoning, radical pelvic surgery, surgery on the rectum and prostate and various types of injuries (such as pelvic fractures) represent conditions that affect the peripheral nervous system. All of these have the potential to affect erections and cause varying degrees of impotence depending on their severity.

Multiple sclerosis is a disease of unknown origin that affects the central nervous system of young adults—usually twenty to forty years of age. In the northern United States, there are 40 to 60 cases per 100,000 people; in the southern states, there are 6 to 14 cases per 100,000 people. The disease is almost twice as common in women as in men.

Men with multiple sclerosis (MS) have plaques or scars in the brain and spinal cord that cause impotence in a fair percentage of cases—an estimated 25 to 45 percent. The longer a man has had MS and the younger he was when he contracted the disease, the more likely he is to become impotent.

Unfortunately, the impotence that results from multiple sclerosis tends to be progressive, even though other symptoms of the disease may undergo remission and relapse.

MS patients can successfully use penile injections or undergo penile implant surgery to restore their erectile function. Partners of MS patients often do the penile injections if the man's hands are weakened by the disease.

Of all the neurological disorders that cause impotence, most is known about the erection problems caused by *spinal-cord injury*. The vast majority of spinal-cord injuries are caused either by compression fractures or dislocation of the vertebrae.

In the United States, there are approximately 7,500 cases of serious spinal-cord injury every year, most of them the results of motor vehicle accidents, diving accidents, gunshot wounds and stab wounds.

Overall, 75 percent of patients with spinal-cord injuries lose some erectile function, usually because the injury interferes with the ability of smooth-muscle tissue to relax.

We have treated numerous patients with neurologically caused impotence, including many with spinal-cord injuries. In the past, clinicians treating spinal patients often ignored their sexual rehabilitation. This is now changing, and it is relatively common for clinical teams to include an individual specially trained in sexual counseling and rehabilitation of spinal patients.

Erections depend not only on signals passing back and forth between the penis and the spinal cord, but also between the spinal cord and the brain. If the nerves between the spinal cord and the penis are intact, then direct stimulation of the penis will cause it to become erect.

However, it also appears necessary for the brain to communicate with the relevant nerves in the spinal cord in order for the penis to *stay* erect. In ways that are not yet understood, these signals from the brain trigger the spinal cord to keep the smooth-muscle tissue of the penis relaxed. Many spinal patients have the capacity for an erection—what they lack is the normal ability to *keep* it erect.

As you might expect, the more complete the neurologic injury, the greater the likelihood that potency will be adversely affected. An injury that involves a total severing of the spinal cord, resulting in complete paralysis and loss of sensation below the severance, is more likely to affect potency than a partial severing of the cord, in which case the patient maintains some nerve function below the site of the spinal-cord injury. Patients whose injuries are in the higher portions of the spinal cord, in the neck and upper back areas, find their erectile function less affected than those with injuries lower down, even though those with higher injuries have more paralysis and loss of sensation overall.

In some spinal patients, especially ones whose injury is high on the spinal cord, sexual excitement can increase blood pressure, decrease heart rate, cause facial flushing and spasms of the pelvis and leg, or result in bladder or bowel emptying. Some of these conditions can be managed with appropriate medication and by emptying the bowels and bladder prior to sexual activity.

-------- ◆ --------

Spinal injuries are so varied that one case can't present all of the possible combinations of problems and treatments, but I'd like to give you an insight into how one spinal patient responded to his impotence.

When Carl first came to see me, he was a thirty-eight-year-old *paraplegic* — paralyzed from the waist down — as a consequence of an automobile accident at the age of twenty-two. He was married and lived in New Mexico, where he successfully managed a gallery specializing in Indian art. In late 1984, he happened to view a nationally televised interview I had given on the topic of impotence and how the recently developed penile injections could benefit patients with nerve damage.

Carl and his wife Suzy flew to Boston to see if self-injection therapy could help him. Carl had the use of his hands, which meant he could inject himself. During Carl's initial interview he told me that his erections didn't get very rigid and were poorly sustained.

Carl's physical examination revealed that he had virtually no sensation in his penis, although he did have some sensation in his pubic area. He wanted to have a sexual relationship with his wife in order to provide sexual satisfaction for her, as well as to experience the emotional aspects of intercourse and whatever physical sensations remained in his pubic area. An ultrasound test showed that he had a normal supply of arterial blood flowing through his penile arteries. Carl wished to avoid a penile implant if possible. He was eager to try self-injection therapy and agreed to remain in Boston until he was able to inject himself successfully with the medication.

The first test dose of medication for Carl was a small volume, 0.10 milliliters (ml), of papavarine and phentolamine. His penis quickly became erect — and stayed that way for two hours. Carl and his wife were beside themselves with excitement. Years of sexual anxiety, frustration, embarrassment and fear were coming to an end. Suzy burst into tears; he held her hand, sitting in his wheelchair with a stunned expression on his face. Carl's dosage was eventually adjusted downward to 0.05 ml (an extremely small dosage) as a precaution against priapism (see pages 120 and 159). My last sight of him that initial visit was as he and his wife entered the elevator to leave the clinic, eager to get back to New Mexico. "Suzy and I have got a lot of catching up to do," he said, waving goodbye.

Every year I get a Christmas card from Carl and Suzy. He continues to use self-injection therapy—it's now over four and a half years—with great success.

LOW TESTOSTERONE AND OTHER HORMONAL DISORDERS

It is difficult to identify the true incidence of impotence due to hormonal problems. Various studies place the figure at anywhere from 5 to 35 percent.

In 1849, the critical role of hormones in sexual function was demonstrated when castration was found to eliminate the sex drive of a rooster, and surgical restoration of the rooster's testicles revived his dormant sex drive. In 1889, it was shown that extracts of animal testicles injected into elderly impotent men restored their erections. Ever since then, hormones have played an important—if sometimes overstated—role in the research, diagnosis and treatment of men with erectile problems.

While disorders that affect potency may exist in the regulation of the hormone *prolactin* and of *thyroid* hormone, the most frequently studied hormonal disorder related to impotence is the problem of inadequate *testosterone*. An inadequate supply of testosterone can result from a host of causes, including congenital abnormalities involving the testicles, genetic syndromes, drug therapy, exposure to toxins, radiation or problems with the brain centers that regulate hormone production—the *pituitary gland* and the *hypothalamus*.

At times in the history of medicine, the role of testosterone in sexual function has been exaggerated, as I mentioned in chapter 1. But, occasionally, it is the important factor in causing impotence.

The first clue that impotence may be associated with low testosterone levels is decreased libido—a diminished sexual drive. Evaluation for impotence associated with low testosterone begins with blood tests to measure testosterone levels. Repeat blood tests are usually performed if the first ones are abnormal. If necessary, more sophisticated tests can be administered by an endocrinologist and evaluated in combination with studies of nocturnal erection patterns and blood-pressure readings of the penis during erection.

Richard first came to our clinic three years ago, when he was fifty-two years because he was impotent and because "my wife sent me." It's quite common to hear men with a low sex drive assign responsibility for their visit to a spouse or lover–in contrast to an impotent man with a high sex drive, who spends a lot of time vividly expressing his frustration with his inability to achieve erections.

Richard had not had intercourse in several years–moreover, he had no desire to resume sexual activity. He explained that he had once been quite active, having intercourse three times per week for years. He denied ever having had mumps, exposure to radiation or testicular trauma, all of which can affect testosterone production. He did have a history of hypertension and of moderate-to-heavy alcohol consumption–two to three highballs each evening for over two decades.

Richard still had occasional morning erections. His flaccid blood-pressure measurements and neurological testing all proved normal. However, his hormonal screening, a blood test, revealed an abnormally low testosterone level. We referred him to the clinic's endocrinologist, who performed several additional blood tests. He confirmed Richard's abnormally low testosterone level, attributing it to a testicular abnormality.

The endocrinologist suggested that Richard forego his daily highballs, informing him that some studies indicate heavy drinking can cause testicular damage. He also prescribed intramuscular injections of testosterone every four weeks. Richard would have preferred an oral medication, but oral testosterone is less effective than intramuscular injections and has a well-documented association with toxic side effects on the liver.

Richard had heard that hormone treatments increased women's chances of developing certain cancers. He expressed concern that his testosterone treatment might put him at risk for prostate cancer. To date, no study has shown that testosterone supplements cause cancer of the prostate. If, however, a prostate tumor is already present, testosterone supplements may increase the rate of the tumor's growth. Since a rectal and ultrasound examination uncovered no signs of cancer in Richard, we considered the treatment safe for him. Annual exams of his prostate–both rectally and with ultrasound–have showed no abnormalities. He has noticed some weight gain, due to retention of fluid and sodium, an occasional side effect of this treatment, but by restricting his intake of salt, he is able to manage the weight problem.

Richard has rediscovered his potency and an interest in sex since starting testosterone treatment. He has become sensitized to his level of testosterone, aware that when his sexual interest and overall drive decline, he needs his intramuscular injection.

PRIAPISM

The term *priapism* derives from the Roman god *Priapus,* a god of hunting, fishing, agriculture, fertility, male sexuality and, perhaps most appropriately, excess.

Priapism refers to a prolonged penile erection that is not associated with sexual desire. It occurs when the penis fails to "turn off" its storage or filling mechanisms. Problems with the storage mechanism are more frequent than problems with the filling mechanism.

Priapism, which has been thought of as a rare condition, is increasing in frequency due to the use of self-injection therapy for impotence. It has been reported to occur in some 2 to 15 percent of patients receiving penile injection therapy, usually during the period when their dosage is first being determined. (For self-injection patients on a regular, predetermined dosage, the incidence of priapism drops to less than 1 percent.)

Some patients and even some colleagues of mine joke about patients who have the unfortunate condition of priapism. "I wish I had his problems," is the standard response. "What's he drinking, doc? Make mine a double!" or "How about we bottle what's circulating in his bloodstream!"

Priapism, however, is no joking matter. Left untreated, it may result in impotence. As you'll see, we've had several patients whose lives have been made truly miserable by priapism.

Medical conditions and drugs have been associated with the triggering of the onset of a priapistic erection, but in only about half the cases are there obvious identifying factors that can be linked to the onset of the condition. Trauma (injury) to the penis can result in priapism. Medications such as antipsychotics, antidepressants, antihypertensives and drugs used to inject the penis for the treatment of impotence, such as papaverine, have been associated with priapism.

A host of medical conditions has also been implicated in priapism. Neurological disorders, which include brain aneurysms, herniated lumbar discs, epilepsy and neck injuries have been associated with priapism. Blood disorders associated with high blood viscosity ("stickiness" or thickness), such as sickle-cell disease, leukemia or multiple myeloma, have all been associated with the development of priapism, as have intravenous feedings containing fat emulsions.

Storage priapism. In a healthy person, the smooth-muscle tissue in the penis's erection chambers relaxes only during sexual arousal and during certain phases of the sleep cycle. If it remained relaxed all the time, men would be in a constant state of erection—which is what happens in a man with storage priapism.

This relaxation of the smooth-muscle tissue may be occurring because some nonsexual factor is acting directly on the smooth-muscle tissue, causing it to relax, or because something is interfering with the body's mechanisms that return the smooth-muscle tissue to its normal state of contraction.

Urologists haven't positively identified these factors. A working hypothesis is that certain drugs may act directly on the smooth-muscle of the penis, causing it to relax; and certain abnormal neurological states may cause the nerves of the penis to relax the smooth-muscle tissue even when there is no sexual stimulation.

Yet another possibility involves the cells lining the lacunar spaces in the erectile tissue. Abnormal blood conditions associated with high blood viscosity may trigger these cells to induce and then to prolong smooth-muscle relaxation. Genetic factors may also be involved in the development of priapism (see box, page 162).

When the storage mechanism is continuously activated, the priapistic erection may become a genuine medical emergency. The inability to drain any blood from the penis during the erection can reduce artery blood flow to the erection chambers (corpora cavernosa) to dangerously low levels. This disorder may prevent any fresh arterial blood from entering the erection chambers.

The penis begins to feel pain as the supply of oxygenated blood to the erection chambers is cut off. Eventually, tissue begins to die. Scarring results from the damaged erectile tissue and then interferes, in many cases permanently, with the ability of the penis to become erect.

Blood circulation through the erection chambers needs to be restored as soon as possible once storage priapism has developed. Permanent damage to the erection tissue has been documented after twelve hours of a priapistic erection.

Treatment of storage priapism involves: identifying an offending drug (if there is one) and discontinuing its use; identifying and, if possible, correcting an abnormal neurological or blood condition; and, in all cases, immediately establishing drainage of blood from the erection chambers and thereby allowing fresh arterial blood to enter the erectile tissue.

The physician may drain blood directly from within the erection chambers. An alternative is to inject the erection tissue with a drug to induce contraction, which will cause lower resistance to venous drainage and induce blood to flow away from the penis. If neither of these measures establishes drainage from the erection chambers, emergency surgery may be needed. *We specifically instruct men on the self-injection program to contact their doctor within four hours of a prolonged erection to avoid the problem of storage priapism.*

Filling priapism. Priapism may also rarely occur because the filling mechanism is persistently activated. This is an unusual reason for priapism and was first recognized as a side effect of early penile revascularization surgeries. In those cases, a new artery was connected directly to the erection tissue, providing unregulated amounts of fresh arterial blood to the erection chambers. Today, the new artery is connected to an existing artery of the penis, thus avoiding the excessive unregulated filling (see illustration, page 82).

Filling priapism is now primarily caused by "blunt perineal trauma"—i.e., a blow to the groin area—or penile trauma. The trauma lacerates an artery, resulting in persistent bleeding into the erection tissue. Since the storage mechanism is not activated, the blood *is* able to flow out of the erection chambers, so filling priapism does not choke off the blood supply to the erection chambers in the same way that storage priapism does. It is therefore not as dangerous.

Treatment of filling priapism aims at stopping the erection artery from bleeding. A radiologist who specializes in arteriography of the penis may be called in. He injects a small amount of the patient's own clotted blood directly into the bleeding artery, which then causes the bleeding artery itself to clot.

———— ◆ ————

Fred, a twenty-one-year-old college student, developed storage priapism while traveling to Europe last summer. He had none of the known risk factors for developing priapism, such as neurological or blood problems, and he took no oral or injectable medication.

Of note, Fred had a history of easily being able to sustain an erection for intercourse for over one hour without much stimulation. Following ejaculation and orgasm, he had been quickly able to attain a second erection. This history is common in patients who develop priapism without any history of disease or medication (see box, page 162). Fred commonly awoke with a firm morning erection, which usually lasted through urination. This forced him into difficult positions in order to be sure of hitting the toilet bowl.

Fred's first priapistic erection began when his morning erection did not disappear, but rather persisted throughout the day, evening, night and the following morning. Needless to say, he slept little that night. Fred was extremely embarrassed by the prolonged erection—a factor common to virtually all patients with priapism, which often accounts for their delay in seeking medical help. The erection lasted over thirty-six hours, and despite the pain, Fred never did seek medical help.

Over the next few days, the erection slowly subsided. During the subsequent six months, Fred was unable to achieve any erections,

Priapism and Impotence—
Two Sides of the Same Coin?

Some men develop storage priapism for unknown reasons. They don't have any of the diseases or medical conditions usually associated with the problem. Nor are they taking any of the drugs that are traditionally known to feature priapism as a complication.

What, then, is going on?

One fascinating possibility is that these men are just a little bit different from the rest of the male population. Genetic variation allows for vast differences among us, while still adhering to the basic human blueprint. These variations exist not only in the obvious ways like skin and hair color, but also at the microscopic level of nerve and cell interactions. One example of this variation is our differing abilities to metabolize cholesterol.

Genetic factors may be important in men who develop priapism for unknown reasons. In interviewing men with this problem about their sex histories, I've found that before the onset of priapism, they usually achieved and sustained erections extremely easily. This held true even after intercourse, when most men must wait a certain period of time before again achieving an erection.

There may exist an underlying, still unknown, biochemical variation in the way that smooth-muscle tissue, nerves or the endothelial cells that line the blood vessels within the erection tissue interact (see illustration, page 13).

It may be that, in some men, the biochemical variation results in constantly *relaxed* smooth-muscle tissue in the penis, and therefore a nearly constant state of erection—priapism. In others, the abnormality may result in constantly *contracted* smooth-muscle tissue, and a nearly constant state of flaccidity—impotence.

whether masturbating, having sex with a partner or during sleep. This caused him tremendous anguish and frustration.

Then, over a period of three days, he noticed the development of an erection. Although somewhat pleased, Fred noticed that on the fourth morning, the erection was very hard, persisted into late morning, and he developed pain again in his penis. This time, however, he sought medical attention. He received an injection of an adrenaline-like drug into the penis with immediate resolution of the erection and of the pain.

The next morning, however, the same priapistic erection developed and lasted three days. Fred now has the unusual problem of recurrent priapism, which worsens if he lies down. He awakens each morning with a painful priapistic erection. He cannot go to classes in the morning until the erection disappears, which it does if he runs or jogs. By exercising, he is probably activating the adrenaline-like nerves that cause smooth-muscle contraction in the penis. If he sleeps longer than six hours or has intercourse, his condition becomes worse. The erection will last indefinitely.

Under our close supervision, he is able to lead a more normal life by injecting his penis with drugs that temporarily reduce the erection. We are considering surgery that would establish temporary drainage from the erection chambers to the chamber surrounding the urinary passageway. Our dilemma in treating Fred is to maintain a balance between allowing him to lead a more normal life, while preserving his capacity for intercourse.

———— ◆ ————

Another patient, Howard, is a thirty-eight-year-old gastroenterologist whom I treated for filling priapism. He is, in fact, the first patient I have ever treated with this problem.

Howard and his wife went to a play one evening, and they sat in the last row of the local theater. At the end of the performance, Howard noticed long lines forming in the aisles on either side of his row, preventing his quick departure from the theater. As he was in the last row, he decided to jump over his seat. Unfortunately, he didn't clear the backrest and landed with his full weight on his crotch. Howard experienced severe pain that took hours to disappear.

On awakening the next morning, Howard noticed that his penis, although flaccid, was slightly fuller than usual. Over the next several days, his penis gradually increased in size. By the third morning, it was fully erect and pulsating. Howard wasn't in pain, but as a doctor, he knew about the long-term consequences of priapism and was too worried to go to his office. Instead, he came to the clinic and asked me to see him.

Howard had no risk factors for the development of priapism except for his recent perineal trauma. He received an adrenaline-like medication in his erection chambers on several occasions over the next few days to treat the priapism, and ultimately underwent surgical drainage, but despite everything, the erections always returned. Howard and his wife were extremely anxious and exhausted by the prolonged, seemingly endless ordeal of failed treatments and a persistent erection.

Finally, after seven days of a full but painless erection, Howard underwent an arteriogram (see box, page 78). This X-ray evaluation is not usually performed on potent men, but the situation was getting somewhat desperate. We hoped the study would confirm our suspicion that a bleeding artery could be causing Howard's priapism. We also hoped the arteriogram would give us its location.

The study revealed bleeding from an erection artery directly into the erection tissue, right at the spot where he'd landed on the theater seat. We drew 3 milliliters of Howard's own blood from a vein in his arm. The blood was allowed to clot, and the clot was then injected directly into the bleeding penile artery. His erection started to dramatically disappear right then and there in the X-ray suite. A follow-up X ray confirmed that the bleeding had stopped. Howard and his wife were elated. They could go on with their lives; he most likely would recover completely in time.

With filling priapism, there is no shut-off of arterial blood flow and therefore no pain with the prolonged erections. There is no obvious long-term tissue damage. It is now one and a half years since Howard's priapism. Within three months he completely regained the erectile capability he possessed prior to his injury. Howard may one day experience the delayed impotence problems associated with perineal trauma, such as problems with filling and storage, but at the present time he is functioning normally.

CANCER AND SEXUAL FUNCTIONING

Over the years, the treatment of cancer has come to rely on earlier diagnosis and earlier, more aggressive uses of chemotherapy, immunotherapy, radiation and surgery. In many cases, this approach means that patients are living longer, but as survival rates continue to climb, doctors and patients are becoming more aware of the need to pay attention to the quality of the patient's life. For many patients, the most terrifying complication of cancer is an accompanying decline in sexual functioning.

Patients should discuss their concerns, desires and expectations with their doctor or another professional, such as a therapist who specializes in such problems. The therapist can dispel any misconceptions a patient may have and focus attention on the problem in a positive, assertive manner, which may result in the patient's seeking treatment for impotence.

———— ◆ ————

The mind-body connection is particularly significant in cancer patients. The diagnosis of cancer and the damage caused by the disease and the treatment (even if the treatment doesn't directly interfere with erectile physiology) both have the potential for lowering a man's self-esteem and giving him a negative image of his body. These psychological reactions to cancer may affect his libido and his erectile response, especially his ability to initiate or sustain an erection.

Some men buy into the old wives' tale that any cancer involving the reproductive organs is connected to promiscuity. Cancer of the prostate, testicle or penis is often a source of shame.

Patients have been known to see these problems as punishment for a real or imagined affair, masturbation, use of contraception or an act of sexual violence. Such patients often go to extreme lengths to identify the past misstep that has "sentenced" them to their disease.

Even patients who don't make a punishment-disease connection will sometimes abstain from sex. Some patients make a secret vow to discontinue all sexual activity in return for continued survival. Others act out of the erroneous belief that they can infect their partner with their disease.

Cancer affects patients of different ages differently. A young man may worry about his inability to engage in intercourse or start a family. In the later stages of life, impotence from cancer may erode the patient's sense of an important long-term bond of intimacy with his spouse.

Cancer patients commonly fear how others will respond to the news of their disease or the effects of its treatment. Disfiguring treatments are a blow to a man's self-esteem and may therefore affect his sexual functioning. Dependence on a *colostomy* or *urostomy* (special devices for eliminating feces or urine through an artificial hole in the abdomen) can be especially devastating.

Not all of the impotence caused by cancer is psychogenic. Cancer or its treatment can directly damage the nerves and blood vessels of the penis. "Radical," meaning wide, removal of the prostate, bladder or lower bowel sometimes damages nerves important to the ability to initiate an erection.

Removal of both testicles may result in a nearly complete loss of male hormone, resulting in a loss of sexual interest. Certain drugs used to relieve pain and for hormonal therapy or chemotherapy may also impair a man's ability to have an erection.

Cancer patients who experience erectile difficulties should approach the problem just like patients without cancer—by beginning with a urological evaluation. A urologist performs the workup described in chapter 1, with the addition of a consultation with the doctor(s) who diagnosed and treated the cancer. The workup may include a detailed sexual and medical history, a physical exam, a blood test to determine the level of testosterone, close questioning about lifestyle factors that could affect potency and other tests as needed. These latter could include monitoring the frequency and rigidity of the man's nighttime erections and, if necessary, more sophisticated testing such as a DICC study (see box, page 102).

———— ◆ ————

Bill, a fifty-nine-year-old sales manager, consulted me because he was having erectile difficulties following prostate surgery for cancer seven years ago. His prostate cancer was discovered in the course of an annual rectal examination. A widower, he had remarried and had been quite active sexually with his new wife until the cancer surgery.

Different types of tumors vary in how quickly they grow. A biopsy revealed Bill's tumor was one of the slower-growing varieties. He had two options for treatment—radical surgery or radical radiotherapy. He chose the former, although he was aware that the surgery carried a high risk of postoperative impotence. Until recently, radical surgery for prostate cancer virtually guaranteed the loss of potency. Nowadays, urologic surgeons have become aware of the vital role that nerves passing close to the prostate play in erectile function. They seek to identify these nerves and spare them if possible during the removal of the tumor and prostate tissue. They have been especially successful in preserving potency in younger patients with tumors confined to the prostate gland.

Bill's surgery went well, but several months after the surgery, he attempted to make love with his wife and his penis refused to achieve more than a partial erection that didn't last long. Naturally, Bill's diminished potency caused him some anxiety, but he and his wife managed to maintain a sexual relationship that did not include intercourse.

After living approximately six years without sexual intercourse, Bill heard about the recent progress being made in impotence treatment and underwent a complete impotence evaluation. His tests showed abnormalities in his erectile mechanism, probably the result of nerve damage during the prostate surgery. We measured his nighttime erections and found them to be infrequent and insufficiently rigid. However, when we gave Bill an injection of papaverine and phentolamine (see page 117), he developed a strong erection.

The impotence that follows radical prostate surgery usually results from damage to the motor nerves that carry signals from the spine to the smooth-muscle tissue of the penis, causing it to relax. Other radical pelvic surgeries, such as cancer operations for rectal or bladder cancer, and spinal-cord injuries, can cause similar "failure-to-initiate" erection problems by interrupting these signals. If the smooth-muscle tissue doesn't relax, the erectile chambers can't fill with blood. No signals, no erection. The papaverine and phentolamine injections bypass the damaged nerves and allow initiation of an erection.

I encouraged Bill to try self-injection therapy. He was anxious to start and experienced his first erections in six years with only a small dose of the drugs. Bill found that self-injections were not difficult to administer. In the year since he started injection therapy, he says the quality of his life has improved dramatically. Happily, he has now also been cancer-free for over eight years.

IMPOTENCE IN TEENAGERS AND THE ELDERLY

In our clinic, the average age of the patients seeking help for impotence is the early fifties. Judging from statistics I've seen from other clinics, I'd say this age is fairly typical for men in the United States. Nevertheless, some of my patients are still in their teens, or are in their seventies and eighties. Both ends of the spectrum raise special concerns.

Teenagers. Teenage impotence appears to be commonly (though not exclusively) the result of blunt perineal trauma sustained, for example, during sports or bicycle riding or an automobile accident. Trauma can injure arteries and induce typical artery blockages. Trauma can also cause tissue stiffness (as in David's case in chapter 5). In both circumstances, the overall penile function is adversely affected. In terms of treatment, the confined nature of the problem usually allows for surgical improvement or cure.

Impotence is extremely difficult for a young person. Young people expect to have firm, hard erections at the drop of a hat—no exceptions. Youth implies virility. At an age when many young people are just becoming sexually active, impotence can be devastating. A young man often expects much more from treatment than an older man. The older man will often have the emotional maturity to accommodate himself to an erection that is sufficient for intercourse, but not as rigid as the erections he got when he was thirteen or fourteen. This isn't usually the case with teenage boys. Their friends have hard erections—and they want the same whether they are sexually active or not.

Other issues can complicate the treatment process. I've had teenage boys come to our clinic without their parents' knowledge. In most cases I have to insist that they share this problem with a responsible family member. On the other hand, I occasionally find parents who push their sons into treatment before the boys are emotionally ready for it.

For most teenagers, the treatment options evoke a profound emotional reaction, usually negative. Many adult men have difficulty grappling with the idea of injecting themselves or undergoing surgery. Teenagers have even more difficulty. In my experience, it's sometimes best to just diagnose a teenager's problem and leave it at that. I let him know that he doesn't have a deep-seated psychological problem and that medical treatment is available — when and if he's ready for it. In the meantime, he can see a sex therapist or counselor experienced in adolescent sexuality. He can also postpone treatment, for years if he wishes. (Often, a high-school student will have his impotence diagnosed but defer treatment until his college years, when he becomes romantically involved with someone.) In my view, delaying this way is often the wisest course of action.

Elderly patients. Elderly patients present different difficulties. As I discussed in chapter 2 (see box, page 25), aging does take its toll on a man's erections. Aging also affects the lubricating ability of a woman's vagina, which poses another barrier to intercourse for the older couple. But, with a willing partner, there's no reason a man can't remain sexually active, including having intercourse, for as long as he wants. For some men, the simple ability to achieve an erection, whether they have intercourse or not, is an important part of their sense of well-being.

If an elderly patient wishes to maintain erectile performance, he can undergo an evaluation and choose from a variety of treatment options. The risks of surgery for the elderly, as well as the reasons for the impotence, usually rule out reconstructive surgery. But few men in their seventies or eighties need — or want — this treatment. Convenience, matched to the less frequent desire for sex, can make many treatments attractive that a much younger man might reject.

An elderly patient may be satisfied with an infrequent penile injection, for example, or the occasional use of a vacuum constriction device (see box, page 169).

———— ◆ ————

When George came to our clinic, he was seventy-eight years old and had been married to the same woman for over fifty years. Until very recently, he and his wife had enjoyed sex once a week and he refused to give up intercourse, saying it wasn't natural to do so. For the last three years, his erections, although initially rigid, had been lasting shorter and shorter periods of time, until it was no longer possible for him to have intercourse.

We evaluated George using noninvasive testing and without doing a DICC study. He wasn't a good candidate for surgery because of his age, so there seemed little point in subjecting him to this invasive

The Vacuum Constriction Device

Vacuum constriction devices (VCDs) depend on suction to develop an erection. The one I sometimes recommend to my patients is composed of a hard plastic cylinder connected by a flexible tube to a hand-held pump (see illustration, page 170). The man inserts his flaccid penis into the cylinder, holding the base of the cylinder tightly against his abdomen so that air cannot enter. The man squeezes the pump with his free hand, emptying air out of the cylinder. The resulting vacuum causes blood to flow into the penile shaft. Most VCDs now come with emergency safety valves that prevent the vacuum from becoming too strong.

When the erection in the penile shaft has been achieved, the man slips a rubber ring off the base of the device over the base of his penis. The ring traps the blood in the penile shaft, producing an erection. The ring may safely remain on the penis for up to thirty minutes. He then releases a lever which admits air into the vacuum, allowing the cylinder to be removed.

The chief advantage of the vacuum constriction device is that it safely produces an erection sufficient for intercourse without recourse to reconstructive surgery, injections or implants. The disadvantages are: the VCD's appearance can be initially daunting—it's large and mechanical-looking; the erection doesn't feel "complete," since only the shaft of the penis fills with blood (the perineal part of the penis usually remains flaccid); accidental bruising of the penis, swelling of the penile skin and difficulty with ejaculation (because the rubber ring compresses the urethra) sometimes occur.

VCDs are excellent for patients when injections, reconstructive surgery or implants are either inadvisable, ineffective or not desired.

testing. We found that George had abnormally low penile blood pressures and had lost some sensation in his penis.

George decided to try using a vacuum constriction device. Although he was initially awkward, he soon mastered the technique necessary for using a VCD. The device enabled him to achieve a satisfactory erection any time he wanted. Occasionally, he experiences

Vacuum Constriction Device (VCD)

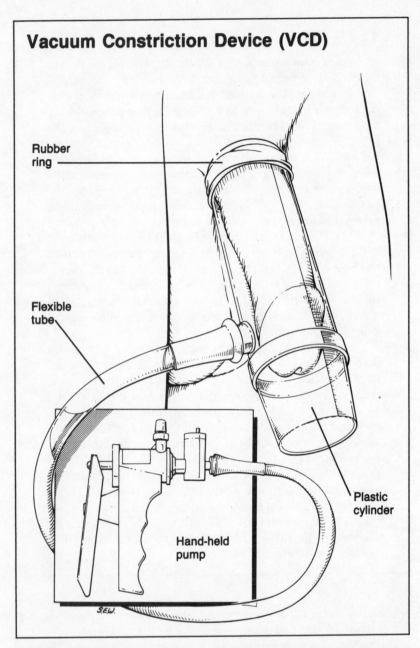

Rubber ring

Flexible tube

Plastic cylinder

Hand-held pump

S.E.W.

With this device, rigidity of the penis is achieved by creating a vacuum-generated negative pressure around the penile shaft, which allows blood to flow into the shaft. A rubber ring at the base of the penis maintains the erectile rigidity after the device is removed.

bruising or interference with ejaculation, but these infrequent complications are more than offset by the device's advantages. George
stops by the office every six months for a checkup. He is eagerly
awaiting the release of an oral medication to improve his erections,
but meanwhile is quite content to continue using the VCD.

MEDICATION-ASSOCIATED IMPOTENCE

Many medications have been reported to cause erectile problems
or reduced sexual drive as side effects. Estimates on the incidence
of medication-induced erectile dysfunction vary, but one physician
reported that 25 percent of patients in a large medical outpatient
clinic had erectile problems as a result of their medication.

The list of drugs that may affect sexual function includes medications designed to lower blood pressure, treat psychoses, depression
and anxiety, cure ulcers, reduce cholesterol, improve heart function
and kill cancer cells. In addition, alcohol, cocaine, marijuana, nar-
cotics and even tobacco have all been reported to lead to erection
problems with prolonged use.

Reports that a particular drug may cause impotence as a side effect must be taken with caution. There are few definitive studies of
any drug's effect on erectile function. Most of the studies did not
include a "control group"— a group of men not taking the drug but
with a similar age, background and vascular risk factors to the men
taking the drug. I don't mean to say that medication-induced impotence doesn't occur— only that it is poorly understood. If you think
your medication may be causing erectile problems, consult your doctor. Changes in the medication or in its dosage may help, but should
not be attempted on your own.

Drugs that are female hormones, called *estrogens,* and drugs that
block the action of male hormones, the *androgens,* have been
associated with impotence. *Cyproterone acetate,* used in the treatment
of prostate cancer, and *cimetidine,* used in the treatment of ulcers,
can decrease libido and sexual interest and result in impotence. *Digox-
in,* used in the treatment of heart conditions, has been associated
with increased levels of estrogen and decreased levels of testosterone
in men and may also cause impotence in some cases. Several of the
anticancer drugs may cause a decrease in libido and sexual activity,
possibly because they also block the action of the male hormones,
the androgens.

Some medications are thought to block the action of the relaxing neurotransmitters that initiate erection in the penis. These drugs
are called *anticholinergics* and include the drug *propantheline bromide,*
an antispasmodic, several *antihistamines* and many of the drugs used
to treat Parkinson's disease.

The class of medications most likely to have an adverse effect on erectile function is the *antihypertensives,* such as *propranolol* and *clonidine*, drugs designed to reduce high blood pressure.

Hypertension affects a man's entire body. If the blood pressure in the artery of his arm is elevated, most likely the blood pressure in the arteries of his penis will also be high. Since antihypertensive medication lowers blood pressure in the arteries of the entire body, it always lowers blood pressure in the arteries of the penis as well. In some men—those whose blood pressure in the arteries of the penis is lower than in the arteries of the arm—this drop in the penile blood pressure may interfere with their ability to have an erection.

In men with normal, unblocked arteries, arterial penile blood pressure is the same as the arterial blood pressure in the arm. Hypertension is associated with the development of blockages in the man's penile arteries, so there is often a gap of 40 to 50 millimeters of mercury in the blood pressure of the arm versus the penis in hypertensive men—enough to cause erectile insufficiency when the hypertension is treated.

It's worth emphasizing that if you're a man with hypertension, then discontinuing your medication is not the answer to your erection problems. Such a step would increase your risk of heart attack or stroke, and even the likelihood of blockages in the arteries of the penis. Over time, these blockages would only widen the gap between the pressure in your penile arteries and the blood pressure in the rest of your body. The hypertension itself might thereby cause a decline in your erections. The best course of action is to see your doctor and ask whether your medication might be adjusted or changed; then, continue taking the medication at the dosage necessary to reduce your blood pressure and see an impotence specialist if problems with erections persist.

———— ◆ ————

The following story shows how one of my patients wrestled with the effects of blood-pressure medication on his erectile function.

Stephan sought help for his erectile problems at the age of fifty-three. He had enjoyed an active sex life, with intercourse four to five times per week, for the last twenty years. He had stopped smoking at age fifty. During a recent physical examination, Stephan had been diagnosed as having a case of moderate hypertension. He was also slightly overweight and had moderately elevated levels of cholesterol. He was put on a standard antihypertensive drug, one that his family doctor had been prescribing for years.

Stephan's arm blood pressure soon dropped to normal levels, but he immediately noticed dramatic changes in the rigidity of his erections. He described numerous occasions when he hadn't been able to achieve an erection and times when his erection wasn't rigid enough for penetration.

Naturally, Stephan was unhappy with these changes in his erectile function. He had been accustomed to having his feelings of arousal translate instantly into a firm erection. With medication, this was no longer the case.

One weekend, however, after forgetting to take his medication, he observed that his erections returned to their previous rigidity. Suddenly he had proof—the medication was causing his erection problems! He immediately returned to his doctor and complained about the drug.

His physician switched him to a new medication, one reported to have less effect on sexual performance. Stephan noticed an immediate improvement in the rigidity of his erections. But, his doctor soon discovered that the medication simply wasn't lowering his blood pressure to safe levels. The dosage was increased, Stephan's blood pressure dropped—and so did his rigidity.

An ultrasound study of Stephan's penile arteries, when his penis was flaccid, revealed lower blood-pressure readings than those in his arm. A subsequent DICC study confirmed a large gap between the readings of his arm and penis. The blood pressure in Stephan's penile arteries wasn't high enough to produce a rigid erection with his "thermostat" set on "low" with the use of antihypertensives.

Stephan joined the clinic's self-injection program and found that a combination of papaverine and phentolamine gave him satisfyingly rigid erections. He has treated his hypertension problem by losing weight and reducing his blood cholesterol levels along with taking his medication. Today, his medication helps keep his blood pressure within normal ranges while the injections allow him functioning erections.

THE FUTURE

As you can see, there are many special conditions, diseases and medications that can adversely affect erections, in addition to the more common vascular problems and injuries covered in earlier chapters. Future medical research is likely to uncover even more physical disorders that can affect erections.

Looking at the history of the field of impotence treatment may make the reader somewhat cynical because, in the recent past, respectable researchers concluded that the majority of erection problems were psychological.

On the other hand, the case histories of the men interviewed in this book and the comments by Dr. Alma Dell Smith demonstrate

the continuing importance of the mind-body connection in the problem of impotence. As future research increases our understanding
of the physiology of sexual functioning, it will remain important
not to lose sight of the psychosexual component of erection problems whether or not organic damage is also involved.

CHAPTER 9

Impotence Prevention and Future Treatments

The last ten years in impotence research and treatment have been the most exciting in the history of the field. Future research promises to open up whole new ways to treat impotence. The continuing spread of knowledge and understanding will soon make impotence just another treatable medical problem rather than the traumatic experience that it has been and continues to be for millions of men. In this last chapter, I'd first like to talk about the ways in which some types of impotence—impotence due to vascular problems and impotence due to certain injuries—may be preventable. While there is still no hard data to support impotence prevention, these suggested steps appear to be logical extensions of our recently acquired knowledge about the mechanisms that underly erection problems. Finally, I'd like to look at some of the exciting ways in which impotence may be treated in the future.

Healthy Lifestyles

In the near future, I think more Americans will recognize that a healthy lifestyle is a major preventive measure against male impotence. The keys will be:

- eating a low-cholesterol, low-fat, high-fiber diet— especially important for men with a genetic predisposition to high blood levels of cholesterol who are able to control their cholesterol levels with diet
- maintaining proper weight
- not smoking cigarettes
- exercising regularly—at least three times a week, but without incurring injury to the crotch area.

The link between lifestyle habits and vascular diseases is widely understood as it affects the heart. Recent research indicates that the same link can be made with the penis.

A study of 440 French men with erection problems found that the impotent men had one or more of the following risk factors— diabetes, high cholesterol levels, high fat levels or high blood pressure. Many smoked. Every impotent man who had two or more of these major risk factors also had low blood pressure identified in the main artery of his penis, a primary cause of failure-to-fill erection problems.

Although there are many good books available that provide guidelines on healthy lifestyles, diet and exercise, I'd like to provide you with some of the information that I give my patients in each of these areas.

DIET FOR BETTER HEALTH— AND BETTER SEX

Over a lifetime, what a man eats may significantly impact on the penile arteries— one important part of successful blood flow and healthy erections. One way to prevent damage to these arteries may be to eat a diet low in cholesterol and saturated fat, especially if you have a family history of high cholesterol or a genetic predisposition to vascular disorders, such as heart disease. Always consult a physician for advice on the best way to manage your cholesterol level. It is important to get blood tests routinely for cholesterol and other fats in the blood. There are now drugs available, in addition to diets, to lower blood cholesterol levels.

The waxy, fatty substance we call cholesterol is synthesized from other substances by the human liver, and is found already synthesized in foods such as eggs and fatty meats like steak and hamburger. Cholesterol is only found in animal products. People need cholesterol for making cell membranes as well as for hormone building blocks. However, the average American man consumes twice as much cholesterol as needed. Cholesterol is a major contributor to the early development of *atherosclerosis*, hardening and narrowing of the arteries due to fatty deposits. When the blood cholesterol level is high, plaques may develop in the arteries and block the flow of blood to the penis.

There are "good" and "bad" cholesterol "carriers"— materials that carry cholesterol through the bloodstream. The material known as *HDL—high-density lipoprotein—*removes cholesterol from tissues. The material known as *LDL—low-density lipoprotein—*transports cholesterol to tissues, such as the arterial walls, where it may accumulate.

Saturated fats (they're called "saturated" because of their chemical composition) also raise a man's cholesterol level. These fats are found in all animal and some plant products. Cream, whole milk, cheese, beef, lamb and pork are sources of saturated fats. A few vegetable products, such as coconut oil and palm oil, contain a large amount of saturated fat as well.

Many products that proudly state they are cholesterol-free contain large amounts of saturated fats—particularly bakery products, since the oils with saturated fat tend to be the less expensive ones. Examples of foods that contain "hidden" saturated fats include crackers, powdered breakfast mixes, commercially prepared cakes and cookies, some dairy substitutes, candy and chocolate bars.

There is almost no need for saturated fat in the diet. The body can make this type of fat from other sources. A man can survive with little dietary saturated fat.

The other kinds of fats are *monounsaturated* and *polyunsaturated* fats. Monounsaturated fats are found in both animal and vegetable products. Originally, researchers felt that these fats did not affect blood cholesterol, but more recent evidence indicates that they may *lower* blood cholesterol levels.

Foods that contain a large amount of monounsaturated fat include olive oil, peanut oil and avocados. These oils should be used in moderation, however, since they are a source of calories. Like saturated fat, men don't need to consume these fats because they can be synthesized from other sources. These fats should play only a small part in any man's diet.

Polyunsaturated fats are found in vegetables and fish. The most common sources of these fats are sunflower, safflower, soybean, cottonseed and corn oils. The body cannot make this type of fat, so it must be supplied by the diet. These fats have been shown to lower cholesterol. However, care should be taken not to overindulge in these fats, since an excess of any fat can lead to weight gain. Men should reduce saturated fats significantly and instead use a little more polyunsaturated fat. Reducing total fat intake may aid in preventing obesity and may help decrease the risk of atherosclerosis and clogged arteries in the penis.

Recent scientific studies have revealed that there may be a beneficial effect from increasing fish consumption. Studies of Greenland Eskimos have demonstrated a low incidence of coronary artery disease and heart attacks in that group, which was attributed to their high intake of fish, seal meat and whale blubber.

Fish have been shown to contain a polyunsaturated fatty acid called *omega-3* that may aid in the prevention of atherosclerosis. In addition, the fat content of fish is very low compared to red meat, making it an excellent meat substitute.

In addition to taking in too much fat, many American men consume two to three times the amount of protein they require. Excess protein from animal sources, such as meats, cheeses and eggs, comes laden with saturated fats and cholesterol. A diet heavy in animal protein adds excess calories and fat and should be considered a high-fat diet, not just a high-protein diet.

A reasonable alternative to a diet rich in animal protein is one constructed using vegetable and grain sources for protein. Vegetable and grain sources of protein do not come laden with fat and cholesterol, so this type of diet is both low in fat and high in complex carbohydrates and fiber. For example, *legumes,* which include soybeans, black-eyed peas, kidney beans, chickpeas, navy beans, pinto beans and lima beans, are the richest source of vegetable protein. Oats, barley and wheat are good grain sources of protein.

A healthy diet should include at least three—and preferably more—vegeterian meals each week. It is neither necessary nor healthy to eat an animal source of protein with each meal.

A number of good books on the market provide sound guidelines to developing a healthy lifestyle. I'd suggest you read *Jane Brody's Nutrition Book* (W. W. Norton, 1981), *Jane Brody's Good Food Book* (Bantam Books, 1987) and Sonja Connor's and William Conner's *The New American Diet* (Simon and Schuster, 1986).

Here are some essentials of dietary advice that every book should cover and that I recommend to my patients:

• Cut back on fast foods, processed or convenience foods and commercially baked goods.

• Drastically reduce the amount of high-salt foods, such as bacon, sausage, frankfurters, luncheon meats, sauerkraut, salted nuts, pickles and salted snack foods.

• Cut down on your salt use in preparing foods.

• Increase your intake of fresh fruits and vegetables. Canned fruits packed in water or natural juice or frozen without sugar may also be used.

• Increase your intake of lightly milled or whole grains.

• Substitute fish, poultry and complex carbohydrates (grains, rice, beans, potatoes, pasta, breads and cereals) for meats, particularly instead of organ meats.

• Broil, roast or steam food; eliminate fried foods.

• Cut down on whole milk, cheese and ice cream.

• Use soft tub margarine, not butter or hard margarine.

• Cook with unhydrogenated vegetable oil, not lard or shortening.

• Cook eggs in their shells, poach or scramble without fat in a nonstick pan. Do not fry.

• Limit intake to three eggs a week if you eat the egg yolks because the yolk contains the cholesterol.

- Try this recipe for scambled eggs: Add one egg yolk to several egg whites. It's surprisingly tasty.
- Try egg substitutes (made from egg whites and artificial yokes) now on the market. Some aren't too bad.
- Steam or cook vegetables briefly in a small amount of rapidly boiling water to help preserve nutrients, flavor and texture, or eat them raw. Raw vegetables are generally more filling than cooked.
- Increase the amount of water you consume to eight glasses of eight ounces each a day. If you are trying to reduce your food intake, sip water between mouthfuls of food to help fill you so you consume less food.
- Try not to eat between meals.
- Follow your doctor's recommendations with regard to your individual needs. (Sometimes medication is used along with dietary changes to help lower cholesterol.)

There is a great deal of evidence that when men change the way that they eat, they can reduce their cholesterol levels. Over a period of time, lower cholesterol levels probably reduce the risk of forming new arterial blockages.

MAINTAINING PROPER WEIGHT

Researchers estimate that about forty million Americans are overweight—20 percent over the ideal weight for their age and height. Being overweight has been linked to coronary heart disease, atherosclerosis, congestive heart failure, angina, stroke and hypertension. Specifically, the evidence suggests that obesity increases fats in a man's circulation, increases cholesterol and may prevent the production of enough HDLs.

A sound diet and regular exercise are the foundation for losing weight and maintaining weight loss. A healthy lifestyle should include constant monitoring of your weight.

SMOKING

The effects of smoking on health were dramatically re-emphasized in 1988 when United States Surgeon General C. Everett Koop argued that cigarettes should be classified as an addictive drug. Although cigarette manufacturers took issue with his claim, the surgeon general's thinking is based on more than twenty-five years of research that indicates how smoking is linked to cancer and other major health problems.

Smoking most likely affects a man's ability to function sexually. Smokers' peripheral arteries are harder, thicker and more clogged than those of nonsmokers. This may be particularly true of the arteries that supply blood to the penis. Preliminary evidence from arteriograms done on impotent men who smoke cigarettes supports this claim.

My advice to my patients is simple — stop smoking. There is no other course to take, for in the long run, smokers are significantly improving their chances of having major problems with their potency.

ALCOHOL AND OTHER DRUGS

Heavy drinking of alcohol, over time, may destroy the ability of many men to make love. Too much alcohol may reduce the production of testosterone in the testicles. Since heavy drinking also impairs liver function, and the liver is responsible for metabolizing hormones, the reduced amount of hormones a long-term drinker does produce can be made ineffective. Heavy drinking may also damage a man's nervous system, which is vital in sexual functioning, as well as cause social and psychological problems that impact on potency. Prolonged use of cocaine and marijuana has also resulted in erection problems.

My advice to patients is simple: Do not drink excessively and do not use illicit drugs.

EXERCISE

It is now accepted medical practice that a proper level of physical fitness should be maintained to enjoy a healthy and happy life. Numerous studies have confirmed the relationship between cardiovascular disease and lack of exercise — the more consistently a person exercises in moderation, the lower the risk of heart attack. Emotional and psychological well-being also improve with regular exercise. Over the past fifteen years, the number of Americans engaged in running, jogging, walking and aerobic exercises has increased greatly. Americans appear to be taking this advice about exercise seriously.

Research also shows that a proper diet must be coupled with exercise. Overweight people actually eat less per pound of body weight than do thin people! If a patient of mine stresses diet and underemphasizes exercise, the result is usually only short-lived weight loss. To attain and maintain an ideal weight, exercise must become an important element in a healthy lifestyle.

The basic questions my patients ask me about exercise are what kind and how much. The types of exercise a man undertakes are extremely important. A sound physical fitness program should promote the following:

• cardiovascular efficiency — the adaptive responses of the heart to exercise

• muscle strength—the ability to accomplish an activity against a specified resistance without injury

• muscle endurance—the ability of a muscle to respond repetitively for a specified period of time

• flexibility—the elasticity of a muscle group and the effective use of the muscle group throughout its maximum range of motion.

Many of the men I see have occupations that involve minimal physical activity. Such men may also avoid exercise, smoke and drink too much and eat the wrong foods. If you are not in good physical condition, you cannot initially undertake an exercise activity with a high energy cost, such as swimming, jogging, basketball, skiing or my favorite—ice hockey. You need to select a less demanding exercise with a low or moderate energy cost, such as walking, gardening or golf. As your physical condition improves, you can move to more demanding activities.

———— ♦ ————

As a general rule, I recommend that every man can start improving his overall health, and thus his sexual functioning, by walking. I like walking for the following reasons:

• It benefits your heart. Like any muscle, the heart needs exercise, and walking is an ideal exercise. Since your heart rate increases during your walk, your heart becomes stronger and your chances of future cardiovascular problems decrease.

• Walking, like all exercise, improves muscle tone. Without good muscle tone, when you lose weight, your skin becomes flabby.

• Walking expends energy. While a half-hour walk will not burn an enormous number of calories, it burns some energy. If you cover a mile or so in a half hour, you'll expend between 100 and 120 calories. This adds up to a weight loss of ten pounds a year if you don't increase the amount of food you take in.

• Walking tends to reduce appetite and therefore food intake, during the walk and for several hours after.

• Walking, unlike biking or other sports involving straddling your perineum over a hard object, will not injure the crus (hidden part of the penis).

• Walking costs very little—a good pair of walking shoes is all that you need—and you can do it alone, although it can be equally enjoyable if a companion joins you.

The best way to start a walking program is to begin in moderation and keep to a daily schedule. Each week, add five more minutes to the daily walk, so that if, in the first week, you are walking ten minutes per day, you will be walking fifteen minutes per day in the second week, twenty minutes per day in the third week, and so on until thirty minutes per day is reached. Thirty minutes daily is sufficient until you feel fit enough either to walk for a longer period or engage in something more vigorous.

There are a number of books on the topic of walking. I recommend you read *Fitness Walking* by Robert Sweetgall with James Rippe, M.D., and Frank Katch, Ed.D. (Perigee Books, 1985). This is a comprehensive book for those who wish to expand their walking program eventually to the level of vigorous exercise. It answers all the important questions you may have about walking.

Protection from Injury

Many of the impotent men I see have had severe physical damage of the groin area because of sports-related injuries (karate is a good example) or because of damage done while riding bicycles, motorcycles or horses. Studies indicate that such activities as bike riding and karate, as well as accidents in which the perineum comes in contact with hard objects, may injure arterial circulation to the penis or injure the storage mechanism of the penis (see illustration, page 21). It is unclear how much injury is necessary to cause serious damage. However, it's prudent to do as much as you can to avoid injuries to the crotch area.

Many men have bought the myth that they are protected because they wear athletic supporters. Unfortunately, these devices protect only the testicles, not the hidden portion of the penis, the crus (see illustration, page 11), or the blood circulation to the penis.

In the near future, I am looking forward to the development of devices that will enable men to provide themselves with adequate protection when they are engaged in sports or other physical activities. In the meantime, men should keep their weight on their buttocks, not their crotches, while riding a bicycle, motorcycle or horse and should consider getting a two-sided, padded bicycle seat. I advise my patients to avoid sports or other activities where a high probability of groin injury is possible.

Future Treatments for Impotence

In the coming years, there are a number of interesting prospects for the treatment of impotence that I'd like to share with you.

Angiodilation to unblock arteries. Doctors are now treating blocked arteries in other parts of the body, such as those leading to the heart, by stretching them through a process called *angiodilation*, dilation of blood vessels. There may also be an interesting role for this procedure in dealing with impotence. So far, it's only being done experimentally.

We may see a time when a man can come in once a year, for example, and get the arteries in his penis stretched. This stretching could be done with a very small *catheter* (tube) with a balloon on its end that would open up the clogged areas of an artery. There are problems with this technique (damage to the arteries of the penis can occur), but doctors are working on perfecting it.

Insertion of "coils" and scarring agents to block off leaky veins. In the future, radiologists may be inserting coils into the veins draining blood from the penis. These tiny coils, inserted by catheter into the veins, will adhere to the walls of the veins and occlude them. With the same catheter technique, radiologists may also be able to inject agents that cause irritation and scarring of the penile veins, which also leads to vein occlusion. So far this technique has only been used experimentally in the treatment of patients with storage problems.

New oral medications. Oral medications may also be used to treat erection problems, including drugs to dilate arteries, drugs to prevent artery blockages (aspirin may be among them) and drugs to block the effects of adrenaline, known as *alpha blockers*. Continued testing should lead us to a variety of oral medications that could be used in certain patients with impotence.

New injectable medications. One day we may be able to inject drugs into the penis that will make the tissues more elastic, improving their ability to expand and store blood during an erection. Such agents may be *collagenases,* enzymes that digest collagen. In the future, we may be injecting drugs into the erection chambers after an injury to minimize the development of scar tissue in that area. New combinations of drugs that relax erection tissue will become available.

Creams and patches. In the future, creams for the penis may be available, or patches with medication may be developed that are similar to the patches that are now applied to the skin behind the ear when a person anticipates motion sickness. A man may be able to spread a cream on his penis that would be absorbed to improve an erection.

New drug delivery systems. Urologists may one day implant a drug delivery system into the penis and inject medications into it every month or two via a catheter. This system would be safer and more comfortable than the present method of injecting drugs directly into the penis.

Better diagnosis, more knowledge. We will do a better job of recognizing and selecting patients who need surgery for their impotence, by using more refined diagnostic procedures and evaluations. With more and more data from future operations, doctors will have more sophisticated and efficient techniques to help impotent men.

I see a time in the not-too-distant future when men will be able to go to any doctor for some basic information about impotence and then be referred, if necessary, to an impotence specialist.

More impotence specialists. Impotence specialists will increase in number, and patients will be referred to these specialists for appropriate sophisticated diagnosis and treatment. Cases of people being lost in the medical maze, misdiagnosed and misinformed, will be events of the past.

A Final Word

We doctors must take advantage of the new science, as Dr. Krane points out in his foreword to this book. The greatest advance of this decade is the appreciation that the state of the penis, either flaccid or erect, can be manipulated by drugs that either relax the erection tissue and cause erection, or contract the tissue and cause flaccidity. Because of this advance, we now have sophisticated tests to diagnose physical abnormalities in the penis's erect state and can prescribe treatments based on these abnormalities. At the same time, though, we cannot forget to treat the "whole person," whose sexual functioning is composed of more than just his penile nerves and blood vessels.

In addition, as Dr. Masters points out in this book's introduction, it is important that the field of impotence treatment achieve professional maturity. We still have much to learn. In the meantime, patients with erection problems, whatever their cause, need facts and information to make decisions. We hope the next decade will provide this much-needed research data.

In the beginning of this book, I talked about the movie *From the Hip*, which portrayed an impotent man as a wimp, and capable of murder to protect his secret.

As the field of impotence research continues its advance, a whole new script is being written that is bright with promise and hope for all those who are now impotent. It the dream of ending the suffering of so many millions of men and those who love them that has driven me for the last fifteen years and that continues to be the goal toward which I dedicate my work and my life. I hope that any movie about impotence in the future will have a happy ending.

Glossary

Adrenaline—A chemical substance, secreted by the adrenal glands, that causes contraction of smooth-muscle tissue in the erection chambers and blood vessels. See **Noradrenaline**.

Androgen—A class of hormones, primarily testosterone, responsible for developing and maintaining male secondary sex characteristics.

Arteriography—An invasive radiological procedure in which X rays of arteries (**arteriograms**) are taken after an X-ray-sensitive "dye" has been introduced into them. Used for locating sites of arterial blockage, prior to consideration for vascular reconstructive surgery.

Arteriole—The smallest vessel of that part of the circulatory system that carries blood away from the heart. Plays a significant role in the regulation of arterial blood flow.

Arteriole, Helicine—The arteriole that regulates blood flow from the cavernosal artery into the lacunar spaces.

Artery—A blood vessel that carries blood, under pressure, from the heart to the arterioles.

Artery, Cavernosal—Also called the "erection artery." Main artery of the corpus cavernosum. Serves as the primary source of blood flow and blood pressure to the erection tissue.

Artery, Dorsal—The main artery serving the skin of the penis, sometimes used in bypass surgery for impotence.

Atherosclerosis—A blood-vessel disorder characterized by fatty deposits, mostly composed of cholesterol, in the walls of arteries. The deposits act as blockages and restrict the flow of blood to areas normally supplied by the artery.

Autonomic Nervous System—The portion of the peripheral nervous system that regulates involuntary or "automatic" functions such as breathing, heart rate and erection.

Biothesiometry—A noninvasive neurological test measuring the vibration sensitivity of the skin of the penis. One of the diagnostic procedures for evaluating the state of the sensory nerves of the penis.

Bypass Surgery—A vascular procedure used to circumvent an arterial blockage, in order to increase blood flow to an organ.

Cavernosal Artery—See **Artery, Cavernosal**.

Cavernosal Vein—See **Veins, Cavernosal**.

Cavernosal Vein Ligation—Surgical tying off of the veins in the rearmost portion of the penis. Performed in men with impotence who have a problem with abnormal storage of blood during erection. May be accomplished in conjunction with crural plication and dorsal vein excision.

Cavernosography—An invasive radiological procedure in which X rays (**cavernosograms**) are taken of the erectile chambers of the penis after they have been injected with an X-ray-sensitive "dye." When used in the diagnosis of impotence, cavernosography is usually performed when the penis is erect. The test is used to help identify veins involved in abnormal drainage of blood from the penis during erection.

Cavernosometry—An invasive test for measuring pressures in the erectile chambers of the penis. Performed when the penis is erect, the test helps diagnose problems with blood storage during erection.

Central Nervous System—One of the two main divisions of the nervous system of the body, consisting of the brain and spinal cord.

Coil—A mechanical device that is inserted by a catheter into a vein, where it attaches to the wall of the vein, creating an occlusion (blockage). This device is used by radiologists only experimentally to treat failure-to-store erection problems.

Collagen—A protein, often arranged in bundles or fibers, which strengthens tissue.

Corpus Cavernosum (plural: Corpora Cavernosa)—One of a pair of cylindrical erectile chambers that make up the major portion of the penis and participate in the process of erection.

Corpus Spongiosum—Cylindrical structure in the penis containing the urinary tube (urethra), terminating in the glans.

Crural Plication—Surgical tightening of the tunica of the rearmost portion of the penis. Used for the treatment of impotence caused by an abnormality in the erection storage mechanism in the crura (see next definition). May be performed in conjunction with cavernosal vein ligation and dorsal vein excision.

Crus (plural: Crura)—The rearmost portions of the corpora cavernosa, the penis's two large erectile chambers, attached to the undermost surface of the pelvic bone.

DICC—See **Dynamic Infusion Cavernosometry and Cavernosography.**

Deep Dorsal Vein—See **Vein, Deep Dorsal.**

Dorsal Vein Excision—Surgical removal of the deep dorsal vein of the penis for treatment of impotence caused by an abnormality in the erection storage mechanism. May be performed in conjunction with crural plication and cavernosal vein ligation.

Dynamic Infusion Cavernosometry and Cavernosography (DICC)—An invasive series of tests designed to evaluate the interaction of the filling and storage mechanisms during erection.

Endocrinologist—A physician who specializes in disorders of the hormonal system, such as testosterone deficiency.

Endothelium—A specialized layer of cells lining the interior of blood vessels or lacunar spaces. New research shows that the endothelium participates in the control of smooth-muscle tissue surrounding blood vessels.

Erectile Failure—Consistent inability for at least a year to achieve an erection during sex with a partner, masturbation or during sleep.

Erectile Insufficiency—Consistent changes for at least a year in erectile rigidity or sustaining capability during sex with a partner, masturbation or during sleep.

Erectile Physiology—The complex of psychological, neurological, circulatory and hormonal interactions that produces an erection.

Erectile Potency—The ability to achieve and maintain an erection sufficient for intercourse until ejaculation. Potency is a relative term, describing a functional erection. Patients who are potent may nevertheless still have an erectile insufficiency.

Erectile Tissue—Penile tissue consisting of smooth muscle (50 percent), collagen (45 percent), nerves, arteries, veins and endothelial cells. Penile tissue has the unique ability to become engorged with blood, thereby increasing in size and rigidity.

Filling Mechanism—The ability of the penis to provide a sufficient flow of blood, under pressure, to create a rigid, spontaneous erection. Along with initiating and storing, it is one of the three necessary mechanisms of the erection process. Problems with the filling mechanism tend to produce partially rigid, slow-developing erections.

Flaccid—Word describing the nonerect state of the penis, characterized by the absence of rigidity or firmness in the erection tissue.

Glans—The head of the penis, a specialized enlargement of the corpus spongiosum.

Helicine Arteriole—See **Arteriole, Helicine.**

Hydraulic Implant—See **Implant, Hydraulic.**

Implant—An artificial device surgically inserted into the erection chambers to provide rigidity in the penis for the treatment of impotence.

Implant, Hydraulic—A class of implants that relies on fluid-filled chambers to achieve rigidity.

Implant, Nonhydraulic—A class of implants that relies on solid cylinders, rather than the use of fluid, to achieve rigidity.

Impotence—The inability to achieve and maintain an erection sufficient for intercourse until ejaculation.

Initiation—Relaxation of smooth-muscle tissue in the penis. Along with filling and storing, it is one of the three necessary mechanisms of the erection process.

Lacunar Space—The specialized, interconnected, endothelium-lined spaces in erection tissue, surrounded by smooth muscle and collagen.

Libido—Sexual instinct or drive; sexual desire.

Motor Nerves—See **Nerves, Motor.**

Nerves, Motor—Nerves that transmit impulses from the brain and spinal cord to muscle tissue, resulting in contraction or relaxation of the muscle.

Nerves, Sensory—Nerves that transmit sensations, from the skin and other organs to the spinal cord and brain.

Neural Lesion—Any localized abnormality on the neural pathway.

Neuropathy—An abnormal condition resulting in diminished function of the motor and sensory nerves. Neuropathy is commonly seen in alcoholism and diabetes.

Neurotransmitter— A chemical released by nerves to communicate with other nerves or muscles.

NPT—See **Nocturnal Penile Tumescence Test.**

Nocturnal Penile Tumescence Test (NPT)—A noninvasive test involving the recording of various characteristics of sleep erections. Such characteristics may include frequency, duration, circumference changes and rigidity.

Nonhydraulic Implant—See **Implant, Nonhydraulic.**

Noradrenaline—An adrenaline-like substance, secreted by nerve cells and the adrenal glands, which causes the contraction of smooth-muscle tissue in the erection chambers and blood vessels.

Occluded—Blocked, as in "occluded arteries."

Organic Impotence—Impotence whose underlying causation is predominantly the result of physical disease or injury, rather than psychological factors.

Papaverine—One of a group of injectable drugs currently used to induce an erection. Papaverine directly relaxes the smooth-muscle tissue of the penis, thus initiating an erection.

Perineum—In a male, the part of the body between the undersurface of the scrotum and the anus. The perineum contains the crura of the penis.

Peripheral Nervous System—The motor and sensory nerves outside the brain and spinal cord.

Penile Prosthesis—See **Implant**.

Penile Injections—See **Self-Injection Therapy**.

Peyronie's Disease—A pathological condition of the penis characterized by the presence of hard nodular plaques and curvature of the erection.

Phentolamine—One of a group of injectable drugs currently used to pharmacologically induce an erection. Phentolamine blocks the effects of adrenaline, thus relaxing the smooth-muscle tissue of the penis.

Plaque—A hard nodular area of the tunica caused by scarring.

Potency—The ability to achieve and sustain an erection sufficient for intercourse until ejaculation.

Priapism—A prolonged erection not associated with desire. Left untreated, priapism may result in permanent damage to the penis, including impotence.

Prostaglandin E1—One of a group of injectable drugs currently used to induce an erection. Prostaglandin E1, like papaverine, directly relaxes the smooth-muscle tissue of the penis, thus inducing an erection.

Psychogenic Impotence—Impotence whose underlying causation is predominantly psychological, rather the result of physical disease or injury.

Revascularization Surgery—See **Bypass Surgery**.

Self-Injection Therapy—A medical therapy in which a patient is trained to inject the erection chambers of his penis with drugs that cause smooth-muscle relaxation, thus inducing an erection.

Sensate Focus Exercises—A series of graduated exercises designed to reduce anxiety and restore mutual pleasure to the partners' sexual encounters.

Sensory Nerves—See **Nerves, Sensory.**

Sex Therapy—Psychological treatment of sexual dysfunction. Sex therapy, especially since Masters and Johnson, is usually behaviorally oriented and short-term. It typically involves sensate focus exercises, with the participants reporting on their progress to the therapist. If necessary, the therapist may recommend counseling or treatment for other psychological problems that may affect sexual function.

Smooth Muscle—One of the three types of muscle tissue used in the body. Smooth muscle forms the bulk of the walls of blood vessels and the erectile tissue of the penis.

Storage Mechanism—The ability of the penis to store blood in the erectile chambers, thereby maintaining rigidity of the penis during erection. Along with initiating and filling, it is one the three necessary mechanisms of the erection process.

Subtunical Venules—See **Venules, Subtunical.**

Testosterone—The male hormone responsible for libido and the development of secondary sexual characteristics (such as the male voice, hair distribution, fat distribution and muscle development).

Trauma, Perineal—Injury to the male perineum caused by mishap or accident. Often occurs as the result of a fall while playing, riding a bicycle, engaging in contact sports or following a fracture of the pelvic bone, as in a motor vehicle accident.

Tunica Albuginea—The fibrous sheath surrounding the erection chambers of the penis.

Ultrasound—A noninvasive technology for measuring flow through a blood vessel. Used for recording blood pressures in the arteries of the penis.

Urologist—A physician who specializes in the diagnosis and treatment of the genitourinary system.

Vacuum Constriction Device (VCD)—An external device that induces a temporary state of erection in the shaft of the penis through vacuum suction.

Vascular Reconstruction—General term referring to several surgical procedures, often performed together, in order to correct a problem with the filling or storage mechanisms. The procedures include dorsal vein excision, cavernosal vein ligation, crural plication and revascularization (bypass) surgery on penile arteries.

Vein—A vessel that conducts blood, usually under minimal pressure, toward the heart.

Veins, Cavernosal—Veins that drain blood from the rearmost portion of the penis.

Vein, Deep Dorsal—Vein that drains blood from the emissary veins in the shaft of the penis.

Veins, Emissary—Veins that conduct blood from the erectile tissue through the tunica albuginea.

Venous Ligation—General term for a surgical procedure tying off various veins of the penis. Used to decrease venous drainage from the penis during an erection.

Venule—Little vein; the smallest vessel of that part of the circulatory system that returns blood to the heart. Compression of subtunical venules during erection enables the penis to retain or "store" blood in the erection chambers.

Venules, Subtunical—Venules that drain the outer lacunar spaces into emissary veins.

Notes

Suggested Reading

It is not within the scope of this book to provide a detailed list of texts on the subject. The reader is encouraged to go to the library for additional reading. The following represents a list of recent books on the subject material discussed in *The Potent Male*.

Berger, E. and D. Berger. *Biopotency.* Emmaus, Penn.: Rodale Press, 1987.

Brauer, A.P. and D.J. Brauer. *Extended Sexual Orgasm.* New York: Warner Books, 1983.

Brody, J. *Jane Brody's Nutrition Book.* New York: W.W. Norton, 1981.

Brody, J. *Jane Brody's Good Food Book.* New York: Bantam Books, 1987.

Connor, S. and W. Conner. *The New American Diet.* New York: Simon and Schuster, 1986.

Gregersen, E. *Sexual Practices: The Story of Human Sexuality.* New York: Franklin Watts, 1983.

Kinsey, A.C., W.B. Pomeroy and C.E. Martin. *Sexual Behavior in the Human Male.* Philadelphia: Saunders, 1948.

MacKenzie, E. and B. MacKenzie. *It's Not All in Your Head.* New York: E.P. Dutton, 1989.

Mason, T. *Making Love Again.* Chicago: Contemporary Books, Inc., 1989.

Masters, W.H. and V.E. Johnson. *Human Sexual Inadequacy.* Boston: Little Brown and Co., 1970.

Morgenstern, S. and A. Abrahams. *Love Again, Live Again.* Englewood Cliffs, N.J.: Prentice Hall, 1989.

Sweetgall, R., J. Rippe and F. Katch. *Fitness Walking.* New York: Perigee Books, 1985.

Technical Bibliography

CHAPTER 1
IMPOTENCE—THE LAST TABOO

Abber, J. D. and T. F. Lue. "Evaluation of Impotence." In *Problems in Urology* 3 (1987): 476-486.

Bancroft, J. and N. E. Skakkebaek. "Androgens and Human Sexual Behavior." *Ciba Foundation Symposium* 62 (1978): 209.

Fisher, C., J. Gross and J. Zuch. "Cycle of Penile Erections Synchronous with Dreaming (REM) Sleep." *Archives of General Psychiatry* 12 (1965): 29.

Furlow, W. L. "Prevalence of Impotence in the United States." *Medical Aspects of Human Sexuality* 19 (1985): 13-16.

Goldstein, I. et al. "Vasculogenic Impotence: Role of the Pelvic Steal Test." *Journal of Urology* 128 (1982): 300-306.

Goldstein, I. "Overview of Types and Results of Vascular Surgical Procedures for Impotence." *Cardiovascular Interventional Radiology* 11 (1988): 240-244.

Goldstein, I. "Penile Revascularization." *Urology Clinics of North America* 14 (1987): 805-813.

Karacan, I. et al. "Erection Cycle During Sleep in Relation to Dream Anxiety." *Archives of General Psychiatry* 15 (1966): 183.

Karacan, I. "The Dilemma of Diagnosing Erectile Dysfunction." In *Controversies in Urology*, edited by C. E. Carlton, Jr., 99- 103. Chicago: Year Book Medical Publishers, Inc., 1989.

Kinsey, A. C., W. B. Pomeroy and C. E. Martin. *Sexual Behavior in the Human Male.* Philadelphia: Saunders, 1948.

Krane, R. J. "Sexual Function and Dysfunction." In *Campbell's Urology*, edited by P. C. Walsh et al., 700-735. Philadelphia: W. B. Saunders, 1986.

Masters, W. H. and V. E. Johnson. *Human Sexual Inadequacy.* Boston: Little, Brown and Co., 1970.

Melman, A., D. Kaplan and J. Redfield. "Evaluation of the First 70 Patients in the Center for Male Sexual Dysfunction of Beth Israel Medical Center." *Journal of Urology* 131 (1984): 53-55.

Padma-Nathan, H., I. Goldstein and R. F. Krane. "Evaluation of the Impotent Patient." *Seminars in Urology* 4 (1986): 225-232.

Shabsigh, R., I. J. Fishman and F. B. Scott. "Evaluation of Erectile Impotence." *Urology* 32 (1988): 83-90.

Smith, A. D. "Psychologic Factors in the Multidisciplinary Evaluation and Treatment of Erectile Dysfunction." *Urology Clinics of North America* 15 (1988): 41-51.

Snyder, P. J. and D. A. Lawrence. "Treatment of Male Hypogonadism with Testosterone Enanthate." *Journal of Clinical Endocrinology and Metabolism* 51 (1980): 1335.

CHAPTER 2
ERECTIONS

Bancroft, J. and F. C. W. Wu. "Changes in Erectile Responsiveness during Androgen Replacement Therapy." *Archives of Sexual Behavior* 12 (1983): 59-66.

Benson, G. S., J. McConnell and L. I. Lipshultz. "Neuromorphology and Neuropharmacology of the Human Penis: An In Vitro Study." *Journal of Clinical Investigation* 65 (1980): 506-513.

Bett, W. R. "The Os Penis in Man and Beast." *Proceedings of the Royal Society of Medicine* 44 (1951): 433.

Blanco, R. et al. "Cholinergic Neurotransmission in Human Corpus Cavernosum." *American Journal of Physiology* 254 (1988): H468-H472.

De Groat, W. C. and W. D. Steers. "Neuroanatomy and Neurophysiology of Penile Erection." In *Contemporary Management of Impotence and Infertility*, edited by E. A. Tanagho et al., 3-27. Baltimore: Williams and Wilkens, 1988.

Tischer, G. M., M. L. Swain and K. Cherian. "Increased Vascular Collagen and Elastin Synthesis in Experimental Atherosclerosis in the Rabbit." *Atherosclerosis* 35 (1980): 11-20.

Furchgott, R. F. and J. V. Zawadski. "The Obligatory Role of Endothelial Cells in the Relaxation of Arterial Smooth Muscle to Acetycholine." *Nature* 288 (1980): 373-376.

Goldstein, A. M. B. et al. "New Observations on Microarchitecture of Corpora Cavernosa in Man and Possible Relationship to Mechanism of Erection." *Urology* 3 (1982): 259-266.

Gregersen, E. *Sexual Practices: The Story of Human Sexuality.* New York: Franklin Watts, 1983.

Hayashi, K. et al. "Effects of Elastase on the Stiffness and Elastic Properties of Arterial Walls in Cholesterol-Fed Rabbits." *Atherosclerosis* 66 (1987): 259-267.

Hedlund, H. and K. E. Andersson. "Comparison of the Responses to Drugs Acting on Adrenoceptors and Muscarinic Receptors in Human Isolated Corpus Cavernosum and Cavernous Artery." *Journal of Autonomic Pharmcology* 5 (1985): 81-88.

Azadzoi, K. and I. Goldstein. "Atherosclerosis-Induced Corporal Leakage Impotence." *Surgical Forum* 38 (1987): 647-648.

Kwan, M. et al. "The Nature of Androgen Action on Male Sexuality: A Combined Laboratory-Self-Report Study on Hypogonadal Men." *Journal of Clinical Endocrinology and Metabolism* 57 (1983): 557-562.

Lepor, H. et al. "Precise Localization of the Autonomic Nerves from the Pelvic Plexus to the Corpora Cavernosa: A Detailed Anatomical Study of the Adult Male Pelvis." *Journal of Urology* 133 (1985): 207.

Lue, T. F. and E. A. Tanagho. "Functional Anatomy and Mechanism of Penile Erection." In *Contemporary Management of Impotence and infertility*, edited by E. A. Tanagho, T. F. Lue and R. D. McClure, 39-50. Baltimore: Williams and Wilkens, 1988.

Lue T. F. and E. A. Tanagho. "Physiology of Erection and Pharmacological Management of Impotence." *Journal of Urology* 137 (1987): 829-836.

Michal, V. "Arterial Disease as a Cause of Impotence." *Clinical Endocrinology and Metabolism* 2 (1982): 725-48.

Newman, H. F. "Physiology of Erection: Anatomic Considerations." In *Male Sexual Dysfunction*, edited by R. J. Krane, M. B. Siroky and I. Goldstein, 1-7. Boston: Little, Brown and Co., 1983.

Padma-Nathan, H. et al. "Development of an Animal Model of Atherosclerotic Impotence." *Surgical Forum* 37 (1986): 640-642.

Padma-Nathan, H., T. Payton and I. Goldstein. "Treatment for Organic Impotence: Alternatives to the Penile Prosthesis." *American Urological Association Update Series*, parts 1 and 2, lessons 11 and 12, 1987.

Rubanyi, G. M., J. C. Romero and P. M. Vanhoutte. "Flow-Induced Release of Endothelium-Derived Relaxing Factor." *American Journal of Physiology* 250 (1986): H1145-H1149.

Ruzbarsky, V. and V. Michal. "Morphologic Changes in the Arterial Bed of the Penis with Aging: Relationship to the Pathogenesis of Impotence." *Investigative Urology* 15 (1977): 194-199.

Saenz de Tejada, I. et al. "Cholinergic Neurotransmission in Human Corpus Cavernosum." *American Journal of Physiology* 254 (1988): H459-H467.

Saenz de Tejada, I. et al. "Smooth Muscle of the Corpora Cavernosae: Role in Penile Erection." *Surgical Forum* 36 (1985): 623-624.

Sharlip, I. D. "Penile Arteriography in Impotence after Pelvic Trauma." *Journal of Urology* 126 (1981): 477-479.

St. Louis, E. L. et al. "Basketball-Related Impotence." *New England Journal of Medicine* 308 (1983): 595-596.

Torrens, M. J. "Neurologic and Neurosurgical Disorders Associated with Impotence." In *Male Sexual Dysfunction*, edited by R. J. Krane, M. B. Siroky and I. Goldstein, 55-61. Boston: Little, Brown and Co., 1983.

Vanhoutte, P. M. et al. "Modulation of Vascular Smooth Muscle Contraction by the Endothelium." *National Review of Physiology* 48 (1986): 307-20.

Virag, R., P. Bouilly and D. Frydaman. "Is Impotence an Arterial Disorder?: A Study of Arterial Risk Factors in 400 Impotent Men." *Lancet* 1 (1985): 181-184.

Wilson, J. D., F. W. George and J. E. Griffin. "The Hormonal Control of Sexual Development." *Science* 211 (1981): 1278-1284.

Wilson, J. D. and J. E. Griffin. "The Use and Misuse of Androgens." *Metabolism* 19 (1982): 1278.

CHAPTER 3
THE MIND-BODY CONNECTION AND THE ROLE OF SEX THERAPY

Barlow, D. H. "Causes of Sexual Dysfunction: The Role of Anxiety and Cognitive Interference." *Journal of Consulting and Clinical Psychology* 54 (1986): 140-148.

Benard, F. et al. "Systemic Infusion of Epinephrine: Its Effect on Erection." In *Proceedings of the Sixth Biennial International Symposium for Corpus Cavernosum Revascularization and Third Biennial World Meeting on Impotence* 16, 1988.

Brauer, A. P. and D. J. Brauer. *Extended Sexual Orgasm*. New York: Warner Books, 1983.

Diederichs, W. et al. "Sympathetic Inhibition of Papaverine-Induced Erection." In *Proceedings of the Sixth Biennial International Symposium* for *Corpus Cavernosum Revascularization and Third Biennial World Meeting on Impotence* 79, 1988.

Euler, U. S. "Quantification of Stress by Catecholamine Analysis." *Clinical Pharmacology and Therapy* 5 (1964): 398.

Fischer, S. C. and A. D. Smith. "Evaluation of the Impotent Male: A Sex Therapist's View." In *Male Sexual Dysfunction,* edited by R. J. Krane, M. B. Siroky and I. Goldstein I, 185-193. Boston: Little, Brown and Co., 1983.

Golden, J. S. "Behavioral Approaches to the Treatment of Sexual Problems." In *Eating, Sleeping and Sexuality: Treatment of Disorders in Basic Life Functions,* edited by M. Zales, 236- 257. New York: Brunner-Mazel, 1982.

Hengeveld, M. W. "Erectile Dysfunction: A Sexological and Psychiatric Review." *World Journal of Urology* 1 (1983): 227.

Lo Piccolo, J. "Management of Psychogenic Erectile Failure." In *Contemporary Management of Impotence and Infertility,* edited by E. A. Tanagho et al. 133-146. Baltimore: Williams and Wilkens, 1988.

CHAPTER 4
TOM—A SURGICAL SUCCESS STORY

and

CHAPTER 5
DAVID—A TALE OF TWO SURGERIES

Abelson, D.: "Diagnostic Value of the Penile Pulse and Blood Pressure: A Doppler Study of Impotence in Diabetics." *Journal of Urology* 113 (1975): 636-639.

Bar-Moshe, O. and M. Vandendris. "Treatment of Impotence Due to Perineal Venous Leakage by Ligation of Crura Penis." *Journal of Urology* 139 (1988): 1217-1219.

Glina, S. et al. "Surgical Correction of Corpora Cavernosa? Leakage Responsive to Perineal Compression: Late Results." In *Proceedings of the Sixth Biennial International Symposium for Corpus Cavernosum Revascularization and Third Biennial World Meeting on Impotence* 142, 1988.

Goldstein, I. "Arterial Revascularization Procedures." *Seminars in Urology* 4 (1986): 252-258.

Goldstein, I. "Arterial Surgery." *Problems in Urology* 1 (1987): 144-158.

Goldstein, I. "Vasculogenic Impotence: Its Diagnosis and Treatment." *Problems in Urology* 1 (1987): 547-563.

Krane, R. J. and I. Goldstein. "Surgery for Impotency: Prosthesis Implantation and Penile Revascularization." In *Adult and Pediatric Reconstructive Urologic Surgery,* edited by J. A. Libertin, 598-614. Baltimore: Williams and Wilkins, 1987.

LeVeen, H. H. "Vein Graft for Vascular Impotence." *Medical World News* 3 (1978): 73-75.

Levine, F. J., B. L. Gasior and I. Goldstein. "Reconstructive Arterial Surgery for Impotence." *Seminars in Interventional Radiology* 6 (1989): 42.

Lewis, R. W. and F. A. Pauyau. "Procedures for Decreasing Venous Drainage." *Seminars in Urology* 4 (1986): 264-272.

Lewis, R. W. "Venous Surgery for Impotence." *Urology Clinics of North America* 15 (1988): 115-121.

Lowsley, O. S. and J. L. Bray. "The Surgical Relief of Impotence: Further Experiences with a New Operative Procedure." *Journal of the American Medical Association* 107 (1936): 2029-2035.

Lue, T. "Treatment of Venogenic Impotence." In *Contemporary Management of Impotence and Infertility,* edited by E. A. Tanagho, T. F. Lue and R. D. McClure, 175-177. Baltimore: Williams and Wilkins, 1988.

McDougal, W. S. and R. F. Jeffery. "Microscopic Penile Revascularization." *Journal of Urology* 129 (1983): 517-521.

Michal, V. et al. "Direct Arterial Anastomosis on Corporal Cavernosa Penis in Therapy of Erectile Impotence." *Rozhl Chirogy* 52 (1983): 587-590.

Payau, F. A. and R. W. Lewis. "Corpus Cavernosography: Pressure Flow and Radiography." *Investigative Radiology* 18 (1983): 517.

Peuch-Leao, P. et al. "Leakage through the Crural Edge of the Corpus Cavernosum: Diagnosis and Treatment." *European Urology* 13 (1987): 163-165.

Post, H. et al. "Dynamic Cavernosography: Venous Outflow Studies of Cavernous Bodies." *Journal of Urology* 134 (1985): 276-279.

Procci, W. R. and D. J. Martin. "Preliminary Observations of the Utility of Portable NPT." *Archives of Sexual Behavior* 13 (1984): 569-580.

Sharlip, I. D. "Treatment of Arteriogenic Impotence by Penile Revascularization." In *Proceedings of the Sixth Biennial International Symposium for Corpus Cavernosum Revascularization and Third Biennial World Meeting on Impotence* 135, 1988.

Wein, A. J. et al. "Expansion without Significant Rigidity during Nocturnal Penile Tumescence Testing: A Potential Source of Misrepresentation." *Journal of Urology* 126 (1981): 343-344.

Zorgniotti, A. W., G. Padula and W. Shaw. "Selective Arteriography for Vascular Impotence." *World Journal of Urology 1 (1983): 213-217.*

CHAPTER 6
NORM—THE INJECTION ALTERNATIVE

Brindley, G. S. "Pilot Experiments on the Actions of Drugs Injected into the Human Corpus Cavernosum Penis." *British Journal of Pharmacology* 87 (1986): 495-500.

Buvat, J. et al. "Is Intracavernous Injection of Papaverine a Reliable Screening Test for Vascular Impotence?" *Journal of Urology* 135 (1986): 476-478.

Goldstein, I. "Evaluation of Penile Nerves." In *Contemporary Management of Impotence and Infertility,* edited by E. A. Tanagho, T. F. Lue and R. D. McClure, 70-83. Baltimore: Williams and Wilkens, Baltimore, 1988.

Junemann, K. P. et al. "Hemodynamics of Papaverine and Phentolamine-Induced Penile Erection." *Journal of Urology* 136 (1986): 158-161.

Kiely, E. A., G. Williams and L. Goldie. "Assessment of the Immediate and Long-Term Effects of Pharmacologically Induced Penile Erections in the Treatment of Psychogenic and Organic Impotence." *British Journal of Urology* 59 (1987): 164-169.

Lee, L. M., R. W. D. Stevenson and G. Szasz. "Prostaglandin E1 versus Phentolamine/Papaverine for the Treatment of Erectile Impotence: A Double-Blind Comparison." *Journal of Urology* 141 (1989): 549-550.

Levine, S. B. et al. "Side Effects of Self-Administration of Intracavernous Papaverine and Phentolamine for the Treatment of Impotence." *Journal of Urology* 141 (1989): 54-57.

Padma-Nathan, H. et al. "Intracavernosal Pharmacotherapy: The Pharmacologic Erection Program." *World Journal of Urology* 5 (1987): 160-165.

Padma-Nathan, H. and I. Goldstein. "Neurologic Assessment of the Impotent Patient." In *Disorders of Male Sexual Function,* edited by D. K. Montague, no. 7, 86-94. Chicago: Year Book, 1988.

Stackl, W., R. Hasun and M. Marberger. "Intracavernous Injection of Prostaglandin E1 in Impotent Men." *Journal of Urology* 140 (1988): 66-68.

Trapp, J. D. "Pharmacologic Erection Program for the Treatment of Male Impotence." *Southern Medical Journal* 80 (1987): 426-427.

Virag, R. "Intracavernous Injection of Papaverine for Erectile Failure." *Lancet* 1 (1982): 938.

Walshauser, M. and P. Schramek. "Efficiency and Side Effects of Prostaglandin E1 in the Treatment of Erectile Dysfunction." *Journal of Urology* 140 (1988): 525-527.

Wyndaele, J. J. et al. "Intracavernous Injection of Vasoactive Drugs: An Alternative for Treating Impotence in Spinal Cord Injury Patients." *Paraplegia* 24 (1986): 271-275.

Zentgraf, M., M. Baccouche and K. P. Junemann. "Diagnosis and Therapy of Erectile Dysfunction Using Papaverine and Phentolamine." *Urology International* 43 (1988): 65-75.

Zorgniotti, A. W. and R. S. Lefleur. "Auto-Injection of the Corpus Cavernosum with a Vasoactive Drug Combination for Vasculogenic Impotence." *Journal of Urology* 133 (1985): 39-41.

CHAPTER 7
TED—THE IMPLANT OPTION

Beheri, G. E. "Surgical Reconstruction of Impotence." *Plastic and Reconstructive Surgery* 38 (1966): 92.

Bergman, R. T., A. H. Howard and R. W. Barnes. "Plastic Reconstruction of the Penis." *Journal of Urology* 59 (1948): 1174.

Goodwin, W. E. and W. W. Scott. "Phalloplasty." *Journal of Urology* 68 (1952): 903.

Gregory, J. G. and M. H. Purcell. "Scott's Inflatable Penile Prosthesis: Evaluation of Mechanical Survival in the Series 700 Model." *Journal of Urology* 137 (1987): 676.

Krane, J. R. "Penile Prostheses." *Urology Clinics of North America* (1988): 103-109.

Malloy, T. R., A. J. Wein and V. L. Carpiniello. "Reliability of AMS 700 Inflatable Penile Prosthesis." *Urology* 27 (1986): 385.

Montague, D. K. "Penile Prostheses: An Overview." *Urology Clinics of North America* 16 (1989): 7-12.

Pearman, R. O. "Treatment of Organic Impotence by Implantation of a Penile Prosthesis." *Journal of Urology* 97 (1967): 716.

Schover, L. R. "Sex Therapy for the Penile Prosthesis Recipient." *Urology Clinics of North America* 16 (1989): 91-98.

Scott, F. B., W. E. Bradley and G. W. Timmn. "Management of Erectile Impotence: Use of Implantable Inflatable Prosthesis." *Urology* 2 (1973): 80.

Small, M. P. and H. H. Carrion. "A New Penile Prosthesis for Treating Impotence." *Contemporary Surgery* 7 (1975): 29.

CHAPTER 8
SPECIAL CONCERNS

Diabetic Impotence

Ellenberg, M. "Impotence in Diabetes: The Neurologic Factor." *Annals of Internal Medicine* 75 (1971): 213.

Goldstein, I., I. Saenz de Tejada and R. Blanco. "Impotence in Diabetes Mellitus." In *Methods in Diabetes Research,* edited by S. L. Pohl, J. Larner and W. L. Clark, 678. New York: John Wiley and Sons, 1985.

Kolodny, R. C. et al. "Sexual Dysfunction in Diabetic Men." *Diabetes* 23 (1974): 306-309.

McCulloch, D. K. et al. "The Prevalence of Diabetic Impotence." *Diabetologia* 18 (1980): 279-283.

Saenz de Tejada, I. and I. Goldstein. "Diabetic Penile Neuropathy." *Urology Clinics of North America* 15 (1988): 17-22.

Saenz de Tejada, I. et al. "Ultrastructural Studies of Autonomic Nerves within the Corpus Cavernosum of Impotent Diabetic Patients." In *Proceedings of the First World Meeting on Impotence,* edited by H. Virag and R. Virag, 210. Paris: Les Editions du Ceri, 1986.

Saenz de Tejada, I. et al. "Impaired Neurogenic and Endothelium-Mediated Relaxation of Penile Smooth Muscle from Diabetic Men with Impotence." *New England Journal of Medicine* 320 (1989): 1025-1030.

Peyronie's Disease

Devine, C. J. and C. E. Horton. "Surgical Treatment of Peyronie's Disease with a Dermal Graft." *Journal of Urology* 111 (1974): 44.

Fishman, I. J. "Corporeal Reconstruction Procedures for Complicated Implants." *Urology Clinics of North America* 16 (1989): 73-90.

Horton, C. E., R. D. Sadove and C. J. Devine, Jr. "Peyronie's Disease." *Annals of Plastic Surgery* 18 (1987): 122-127.

Nesbit, R. M. "Congenital Curvature of the Phallus: Report of Three Cases with Description of Corrective Operation." *Journal of Urology* 93 (1965): 230.

Smith, B. H. "Peyronie's Disease." *American Journal of Clinical Pathology* 45 (1966): 670.

Van de Berg, J. S. et al. "Peyronie's Disease: An Electron Microscopic Study." *Journal of Urology* 126 (1981): 333-336.

Williams, J. L. and G. G. Thomas. "The Natural History of Peyronie's Disease." *Journal of Urology* 103 (1970): 7.

Willscher, M. K. "Peyronie's Disease." In *Male Sexual Dysfunction*, edited by R. J. Krane, M. B. Siroky and I. Goldstein, no. 8, 87-99. Boston: Little, Brown and Co., 1983.

Neurologic Impotence

Amelar, R. D. and L. Dubin. "Sexual Function and Fertility in Paraplegic Males." *Urology* 20 (1982): 61-65.

Bors, E. and E. A. Commarr. "Urological Disturbances of Sexual Function with Special Reference to 529 Patients with Spinal Cord Injury." *Urology Survey* 10 (1960): 191.

Chapelle, P. A., J. Durand and P. Lacert. "Penile Erection Following Complete Spinal Cord Injury in Man." *British Journal of Urology* 52 (1980): 216.

Goldstein, I. et al. "Neurologic Abnormalities in Multiple Sclerosis." *Journal of Urology* 128 (1982): 541.

Goldstein, I. "Neurologic Impotence." In *Male Sexual Dysfunction*," edited by R. J. Krane, M. B. Siroky and I. Goldstein, 193-201. Boston: Little, Brown and Co., 1983.

Yalla, S. V. "Sexual Dysfunction in the Paraplegic and Quadriplegic." In *Management of Male Impotence*, edited by A. H. Bennett, 181-191. Baltimore: Williams and Wilkins, 1982.

Endocrinologic Impotence

Griffen, J. E. and J. D. Wilson. "Disorders of the Testes and Male Reproductive Tract." In *Textbook of Endocrinology*, edited by J. D. Wilson and D. W. Foster. Philadelphia: W. B. Saunders, 1986.

Lipsett, M. B. "Physiology and Pathology of the Leydig Cell." *New England Journal of Medicine* 303 (1980): 682.

McLure, R. D. "Endocrine Investigation and Therapy." *Urology Clinics of North America* 14 (1987): 471-488.

Pogach, L. M. and J. L. Vaitukaitis. "Endocrine Disorders Associated with Erectile Dysfunction." In *Male Sexual Dysfunction*, edited by R. J. Krane, M. B. Siroky and I. Goldstein, 63-76. Boston: Little, Brown and Co., 1983.

Spark, R. F., R. A. White and P. B. Connolly. "Impotence Is Not Always Psychogenic: Newer Insights into Hypothalamic-Pituitary-Gonadal Dysfunction." *Journal of the American Medical Association* 243 (1980): 750-755.

Priapism

Hellstrom, J. W. G., J. W. McAninch and T. F. Lue. "Priapism: Physiology and Treatment." In *Problems in Urology: Sexual Dysfunction* (1987): 518-528.

Hinman, F. "Priapism: Reasons for Failure of Therapy." *Journal of Urology* 83 (1960): 420-428.

Lue T. F. et al. "Priapism: A Refined Approach to Diagnosis and Treatment." *Journal of Urology* 136 (1986): 104.

Saenz de Tejada, I. et al. "Regulation of Adrenergic Activity in Penile Corpus Cavernosum." *Journal of Urology* 135 (1986): 142-147.

Winter, C. C. "Cure for Idiopathic Priapism: New Procedure for Creating Fistula between Glans Penis and Corpora Cavernosa." *Urology* 8 (1976): 389.

Witt, M. A., I. Goldstein et al. "Traumatic Laceration of Intracavernosal Arteries: The Pathophysiology of Non-Ischemic, High-Flow Arterial Priapism." *Journal of Urology*, in press.

Cancer and Impotence

Glasgow, M., V. Halfin and A. F. Althausen. "Sexual Response and Cancer." *Ca—A Cancer Journal for Clinicians* 37 (1987): 322-333.

Goldstein, I. et al. "Radiation-Associated Impotence: A Clinical Study of Its Mechanism." *Journal of the American Medical Association* 251 (1984): 903-910.

Goldstein, I., M. B. Siroky and R. J. Krane. "Iatrogenic Impotence." In *Male Sexual Dysfunction*, edited by R. J. Krane, M. B. Siroky and I. Goldstein, 125-134. Boston: Little, Brown and Co., 1983.

Schover, L. R. and A. C. Von Eschenbach. "Sexual and Marital Counseling with Men Treated for Testicular Cancer." *Journal of Sexual and Marital Therapy* 10 (1984): 29-40.

Swanson, D. A. "Cancer of the Bladder and Prostate: The Impact of Therapy on Sexual Function." In *Sexual Rehabilitation of the Urologic Cancer Patient*, edited by A. C. Von Eschenbach and D. Rodriguez, 89-107. Boston: G. K. Hall, 1981.

Aging and Impotence

Cerami, A., H. Vlasssara and M. Brownlee. "Glucose and Aging." *Scientific American* 256 (1987): 90-96.

Ellis, W. J. and J. T. Grayhack. "Sexual Function in Aging Males after Orchiectomy and Estrogen Therapy." *Journal of Urology* 89 (1963): 895.

Harman, S. M. and P. D. Tsitouras. "Reproductive Hormones in Aging Men: Measurement of Sex Steroids, Basal Luteinizing Hormone and Leydig Cell Response to Human Chorionic Gonadotropin." *Journal of Clinical Endocrinology and Metabolism* 51 (1978): 35.

Karacan, I. et al. "Sleep-Related Penile Tumescence as a Function of Age." *American Journal of Psychiatry* 132 (1975): 932.

Kinsey, A. C., W. Pomeroy and C. Martin. "Age and Sexual Outlet." In *Sexual Behavior in the Human Male*, edited by A. Kinsey, W. Pomeroy and C. Martin, 218-262. Philadelphia: W. B. Saunders, 1948.

Pirke, K. M. and P. Doerr. "Age-Related Changes in Free Plasma Testosterone, Dihydrotestosterone and Estradiol." *Acta Endocrinology* 80 (1975): 171.

Medication-Associated Impotence

Goldstein, I. and R. J. Krane. "Drug-Induced Sexual Dysfunction." *World Journal of Urology* 1 (1983): 239.

Nagler, H. M. and C. A. Olsson. "Drug-Related Male Sexual Dysfunction." In *Male Sexual Dysfunction*, edited by R. J. Krane, M. B. Siroky and I. Goldstein, 113-123. Boston: Little, Brown and Co., 1983.

Seagraves, R. T. et al. "Erectile Dysfunction Associated with Pharmacological Agents." In *Diagnosis and Treatment of Erectile Disturbances*, edited by R. T. Seagraves and H. W. Schoenberg, 22-63. New York: Plenum, 1985.

Slag, M. F. et al. "Impotence in Medical Clinic Outpatients." *Journal of the American Medical Association* 249 (1983): 1736.

Wein, A. J. and K. Van Arsdalen K. "Drug-Induced Male Sexual Dysfunction." *Urology Clinics of North America* 15 (1988): 23-31.

CHAPTER 9
IMPOTENCE PREVENTION AND
FUTURE TREATMENTS

Brown, G. D. et al. "Effects of Two 'Lipid-Lowering' Diets on Plasma Lipid Levels of Patients with Peripheral Vascular Disease." *Journal of the American Dietetic Association* 84 (1984): 546.

Fripp, R. R. et al. "Aerobic Capacity, Obesity, and Atherosclerotic Risk Factors in Male Adolescents." *Pediatrics* 75 (1985): 813.

Kannel, W. B. and A. Schatzkin. "Risk Factor Analysis." *Progress in Cardiovascular Disease* 26 (1983): 309.

Morales, A. et al. "Oral and Transcutaneous Pharmacologic Agents in the Treatment of Impotence." *Urology Clinics of North America* 15 (1988): 87-93.

Newman III, W. P., et al. "Relation of Serum Lipoprotein Levels and Systolic Blood Pressure to Early Atherosclerosis." *New England Journal of Medicine* 314 (1986): 138.

Talley, J. D. and I. S. Crawley. "Transdermal Nitrate, Penile Erection and Spousal Headache." *Annals of Internal Medicine* 103 (1985): 804.

Valji, K. and J. J. Bookstein. "Commentary: Percutaneous Transluminal Angioplasty in Arteriogenic Impotence." In *Current Operative Urology*, edited by E. D. Whitehead, 280- 286. Phildadelphia: J. B. Lippincott, 1989.

Index

Morning erections, 39
Motor nerves, 115, 154
Multiple sclerosis, 26, 154

N
Nerves, 17, 115, 154
    damage to, 18, 165
    diabetes and, 154
Nervous system, 17
    alcohol and, 180
    autonomic, 17
    central, 17, 154
    detumescence and, 18
    ejaculation and, 18
    erection and, 18
    parasympathetic, 17
    peripheral, 17, 154
    sympathetic, 17
Neurologic disorders, 147, 154
Neurologist, role in impotence treatment, 6
Neurotransmitters, 22, 42
Nocturnal erections, 76
Nocturnal Penile Tumescence Test, 77
Nonhydraulic penile implants, 133
Nonhydraulic penile implants, *illustration*, 134
"Noninflatable" penile implants, 133
Noradrenaline, 47, 102
Number of impotent men, 1
Numbness of penis, 115

O
Oils, 177
Omega-3, 177
One-piece hydraulic penile implant, 137
Oral medications, 32, 183
Organic impotence, 41
Orgasm, 17

P
Pain, after penile implant surgery, 138
Papaverine, 72, 102, 111, 117
Papaverine injections, 83
Parasympathetic nervous system, 17
Parkinson's disease, 154
Partner, penile injections and, 119
Patch medications, 183
Pelvic fractures, 26
Pelvic surgery, 26, 154
Penile blood pressure, 76, 77
Penile implant surgery, 37, 130
    counseling and, 144
    intercourse after, 139
Penile implants, 37, 125
    appearance of penis with, 142
    blood loss during surgery, 143
    complications with, 143
    dissatisfaction with, 144
    erections with, 132, 141
    history of, 132
    hydraulic, 133, 135
    hydraulic, *illustration*, 136
    "inflatable," 133
    insurance coverage of, 143
    interest in sex with, 141
    nonhydraulic, 133
    nonhydraulic, *illustration*, 134
    "noninflatable," 133
    one-piece hydraulic type, 137
    pain after surgery, 138
    penile sensation with, 142
    recovery from surgery, 138
    removal of, 143
    satisfaction with, 141
    sex therapy and, 132, 144
    sexual adjustment with, 144
    surgery to insert, 138
    three-piece hydraulic type, 137

three-piece hydraulic type, *illustration*, 136
    two-piece hydraulic type, 137
    types of, 133
    urination with, 142
Penile injections, 72, 83, 109, 140
    comfort with, 112
    erections and, 117
    Food and Drug Administration and, 121
    partner's reaction to, 119
    priapistic erections and, 120
    risks with, 119
    technique, 112
Penile injections, *illustration*, 119
Penile prostheses. *See* Penile implants.
Penile sensation, penile implants and, 142
Penis
    anatomy of, 10
    anatomy of, *illustration*, 11, 12
    appearance with penile implant, 142
    arteries of, 20
    atherosclerosis and, 40
    clogged arteries in, 177
    numbness of, 115
    self-injection of, 112
    self-injection of, *illustration*, 119
    veins of, 20
Performance anxiety, 47
Perineum, injury to, 101
Peripheral nervous system, 17, 154
Peripheral sensory nerves, 115
Peyronie, François de la, 151
Peyronie's disease, 147, 151
Peyronie's disease, *illustration*, 152
Phentolamine, 72, 96, 102, 111, 117
Physical causes of impotence, 3
Physical exam, in impotence evaluation, 7
Pituitary gland, 157
Plaques, Peyronie's disease and, 151
Polyunsaturated fats, 177
Potency, 24
Prevention of impotence, 40, 175
Priapism, 111, 120, 159, 162
    filling, 161
    genetic factors in, 162
    impotence and, 147, 162
    injury to penis and, 159
    medical conditions associated with, 159
    medications associated with, 159
    self-injection therapy and, 159
    storage, 159
Priapistic erections. *See* Priapism.
Prolactin, 157
Propantheline bromide, 171
Propranolol, 172
Prostaglandin E1, 72, 98, 117
Prostate gland, 16
    cancer of, 166
    surgery of, 16, 154
Prostatic fluid, 16
Prostheses, penile. *See* Penile implants.
Psychiatrist, role in impotence treatment, 6
Psychoanalysis, 48
Psychogenic impotence, 18, 41, 50, 80
Psychological factors in impotence, 3, 40, 80
Psychologist, role in impotence treatment, 6

R
Rectal surgery, 154
Revascularization surgery, 35, 67, 81, 83, 89
Revascularization surgery, *illustration*, 82

S
Saturated fats, 176, 177
Scarring agents, leaking veins and, 183
Scarring of erectile tissue, 105
Scrotum, 15
Self-esteem, impotence and, 74, 85